the

NEW

Fat
Flush

Journal

and Shopping Guide

Also by Ann Louise Gittleman, PhD, CNS

The New Complete Fat Flush Program

The New Fat Flush Cookbook

The New Fat Flush Foods

The New Fat Flush Journal and Shopping Guide

The New Fat Flush Fitness Plan

The New Fat Flush Plan

Fat Flush for Life

Zapped

The Gut Flush Plan

The Fast Track Detox Diet

Hot Times

Ann Louise Gittleman's Guide to the 40/30/30 Phenomenon

Eat Fat, Lose Weight Cookbook

The Living Beauty Detox Program

Why Am I Always So Tired?

Super Nutrition for Men

How to Stay Young and Healthy in a Toxic World

Eat Fat, Lose Weight

Overcoming Parasites

Super Nutrition for Menopause

Beyond Probiotics

The 40/30/30 Phenomenon

Before the Change

Your Body Knows Best

Get the Salt Out

Get the Sugar Out

Guess What Came to Dinner? Parasites and Your Health

Super Nutrition for Women

Beyond Pritikin

Eat Fat, Lose Weight for Kindle

the

NEW

Fat
Flush
Journal
and Shopping Guide

ANN LOUISE GITTLEMAN,
PhD, C.N.S.

Mc
Graw
Hill
Education

New York Chicago San Francisco Athens
London Madrid Mexico City Milan New Delhi
Singapore Sydney Toronto

1 2 3 4 5 6 7 8 9   QFR   22 21 20 19 18 17

ISBN   978-1-260-01208-8
MHID   1-260-01208-5

e-ISBN   978-1-260-01209-5
e-MHID   1-260-01209-3

This book is for educational purposes. It is not intended as a substitute for medical advice. Please consult a qualified healthcare professional for individual health and medical advice. Neither McGraw-Hill Education nor the author shall have any responsibility for any adverse effects arising directly or indirectly as a result of the information provided in this book.

McGraw-Hill Education books are available at special quantity discounts to use as premiums and sales promotions or for use in corporate training programs. To contact a representative, please visit the Contact Us pages at www.mhprofessional.com.

Contents

Introduction

You are the masterpiece of your own life.

—Dr. Joe Vitale

Welcome to your Fat Flush journey.

My hope is that during this time, as your body detoxes, heals, and renews, so will your spirit. Quite simply, please think of this guide as Fat Flush first aid for your soul.

That's because Fat Flush is much more than just a weight loss program. It's a complete lifestyle transformation on all levels that makes you feel so good and makes you feel so good about yourself (your clothes start to feel looser, your energy increases, your cravings diminish, and your skin looks radiant) that you simply choose *not* to relapse into those old habits that don't support your best self.

It's time for you to join the hundreds of thousands of men and women who have fully embraced the Fat Flush lifestyle and experienced a true rebirth of their physical and mental well-being. But you don't have to do it alone.

Sometimes we all need a gentle nudge or a burst of inspiration to keep us motivated, remind us of why we started, or reignite our goals if we've gotten off track. That's exactly what this journal is for and why it's such an important component of the Fat Flush experience. It provides a safe haven or sanctuary where you don't have to take care of anyone but yourself. It allows you reflective time to discover and embrace your most authentic self.

For many of you, this journal may be the only opportunity where, for a few minutes, you get to focus entirely on yourself, reflecting on your progress, celebrating your triumphs—big and small—and being entirely candid with yourself about what areas need improvement.

Journaling is also a tool that works wonders to help you to identify triggers associated with falling back on old habits. It's amazing how helpful it is to see in writing what emotions and challenges you faced during the day alongside what your diet consisted of. Once you've identified these triggers, you can be prepared the next time you face them. For example, if you notice that after high-stress situations, your response is to immediately reach for a comfort food, make sure a yummy but healthy choice is easily accessible for the next time a stressor surfaces.

When it comes to your weight, I'm a firm believer in throwing out the scale—but not throwing in the towel—when you don't see your weight budging. While I provide space for you to record your weight, always keep in mind that as you begin to tone up, your size can decrease while your weight may remain the same. Remember that muscle weighs more than fat. The best measurement of success is your tape measure, which is why I want you to measure yourself once a week.

The *Fat Flush Journal* helps you keep tabs on all the little steps along the way in your personal Fat Flush journey. As the latest research continues to show, it is those baby-step changes that you make day by day in your eating habits that have the longest-lasting effects. For example, many Fat Flushers use phase 1 for periodic detox and cleansing and follow their regular eating programs for the rest of the time. But they integrate their Fat Flush staples—like the daily eight glasses of cran-water—as part of their "normal" dietary regimens.

This journal can help you to identify the unconscious physical and emotional roadblocks to both weight loss and overall health, thus enabling you to fix them and get back in the driver's seat. Once you are back on track, the following sage advice will keep you there: "Nothing in this world can take the place of persistence. Talent will not; nothing is more common than unsuccessful men with talent. Genius will not; unrewarded genius is almost a proverb. Education will not; the world is full of educated derelicts. Persistence and determination alone are omnipotent." This is my favorite inspirational quote of all time, from Calvin Coolidge, the president of the United States.

Keeping this quote on your laptop or on your desk and journaling through the experience should help to take away your guilt and remorse when you deviate from the Fat Flush path. You just get up and dust yourself off and keep on truckin'.

I've included motivational quotes on every day of the journal so that you can find new inspiration each time you write.

Daily journaling can also help to pinpoint where you need to tweak your diet if you have hit a plateau. It can help you to set realistic goals and know when you have achieved them. It can help you get back to your authentic self and regain your personal power.

In addition to the journal pages, I have provided a shopping list to make Fat Flush as convenient as possible on the shopping front. This handy list includes my favorite brands to make your next trip to the grocery store a breeze!

I've also included a vitality and wellness section with my favorite tried-and-true remedies to recharge, relax, and feel truly radiant from the inside out. It's "the cranberry on top," so to speak.

I personally congratulate each and every one of you who is so courageous in striking out to lead a more conscious and balanced life. The time has come for you to start to recognize and acknowledge your own progress in making better diet and lifestyle choices.

Now, welcome to your new Fat Flush lifestyle—and the journey to your most healthy, happy, authentic self.

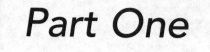

Part One

Part One

Fat Flush Nation

If you want to go quickly, go alone. If you want to go far, go together.

—AFRICAN PROVERB

Fat Flush not only provides a pathway to take your health into your own hands and truly empower yourself. It also invites you into a new, thriving community. We call it the Fat Flush Nation. Found online on Facebook at https://www.facebook.com/groups/fatflushcommunity/, it's composed of an incredibly supportive group of fellow Fat Flushers who are on the journey with you. Share your progress, ask for advice, and connect during triumphs and struggles with this supportive safe place that spans the globe.

Here are the kinds of inspirational posts real-life Fat Flushers share on the Fat Flush Nation.

> This is the only eating plan that eliminated my hip, thigh, and belly fat that have been my constant companion for all my adult years! It also eliminated my hot flashes, cravings—even for my beloved dark chocolate, but amazingly, I don't miss it!
>
> *—Robyn R. G.*

> I fell in love with the Fat Flush Plan because it was so much more than weight loss; there was systemic healing that took place from the inside out.
>
> *—Thesa B.*

> I started the Fat Flush in 1989 with Beyond Pritikin. I've been doing the two-week Fat Flush four times a year ever since! Besides the obvious health benefits and glowing skin, I find that letting go of packaged, processed food in favor of fresh foods has increased my enjoyment of food. My taste buds have come alive; the simplest foods are so delicious!
>
> *—Kay B.*

For the first time since I can remember, my scale is heading in the negative direction. So excited! My emotional gain has been so much more significant than my physical loss. So happy!

—Elizabeth F.

I've been a Fat Flusher since 2002; it's been a life changer. Low cholesterol and blood pressure; little to no belly fat; I sleep well; and have overall wellness. Turning 52 this month. Thank you, Ann Louise.

—Jennifer H. S.

I've lost over 10 lbs. I'm sleeping better, have glowing skin, better digestion, and a clearer mind. My liver and digestive issues are healing. I am becoming extremely healthy! I, for the first time, am confident that I will drop even more because this has become a lifestyle for me. Everywhere I go I'm getting compliments about my healthy glow and smaller size.

—Tami O. C.

I'm so excited! I had to share! Day 5 and I've lost 7 pounds! I finally have the Body Protein to my tasting! I've added Flora-Key, chia seeds, and frozen strawberries—I'm so excited! Delish!

—Tara Ann S.

I've lost 20 lbs., but the best is the inches and that cholesterol down 30 pts, LDL down 20 pts!

—Janice S.

Finished the first two weeks of the Smoothie Shakedown yesterday with a total loss of 12 lbs. and 2⅛ inches off my waist! Struggling to find my appetite, and this is my week-long break of eating 2 meals and 1 smoothie, so going to dig deep to eat enough to keep my metabolism revved up. This plan works!!! :)

—Dawn J.

Excited to share my success story. I lost about 20 pounds when I was in college about 16 years ago, through this incredible Fat Flush program. I remember being an awkward 20-year-old in the original FF message boards!

Fast-forward to moving to SF in my mid-30s, going through a new type of transition period in my career and big move, and gaining 15–20 pounds. I started feeling super lost with dieting and my health. Just feeling completely icky and losing my energy and drive. Nothing had worked in these past 3 years and I have just been steadily gaining more weight and feeling unhealthy and unwell.

Finally, I turned to the one way of eating that helped me through that early adulthood transition period. And I'm glad I did. About 2 months later I am almost at my goal weight! I am so happy to have rediscovered the FF way of life and I can't believe the solution was right there all along. I think for me the big obstacle was the dairy, sugar and the wine. On diets I had been trying, these were still allowed. Once I jumped back to the FF lifestyle, the pounds started melting right off . . . no joke!

I wanted to post here to thank Ann Louise Gittleman for finding a breakthrough program that withstands the test of time, to thank moderator Kathleen for coordinating this group, and to encourage all the ladies in here to keep at it because you will absolutely see results and feel great again. Love you guys! Looking forward to continuing this process with every one of you.

—*Ann M.*

11 days ago I started something I thought would be difficult. It was restrictive, but thanks to Ann Louise Gittleman's diet and book, I lost over 18 lbs. in just 11 days! I feel great and look different!

—*Dwight N.*

Finished first week of Smoothie Shakedown. I lost 5 pounds this week! I try not to focus too much on the scale, but it was a huge psychological boost to break 150. Lost ¾ inches on thigh; other measurements stable, but I haven't been measuring my arms or calves and I can tell that I've lost more there as well. I've also lost more cellulite and am getting excited to see and feel even more muscle definition. Feeling empowered to do this for one more week and also knowing that this is a simple program I can turn to whenever I need a detox and/or reset for cravings and mindset. The journey continues. Hooray and thanks to all of you who post on here—your authentic celebrations and struggles keep me on track. And of course, thanks to Ann Louise and Kathleen and all of our great administrators. :) Have a great day everyone.

—*Kimberly S.*

It has been two weeks since I started Phase 1. After two or three days of headaches, I started feeling good. I have more energy during the day and don't feel sleepy after lunch. I've lost about 5½ to 6 lbs. My clothes, which had been snug and uncomfortable, now fit a little loose and are more comfortable. I am hoping to keep going for a while . . . I would like to lose 25–30 lbs.

—*Janet P. Y.*

Enhanced Wellness Practices in the Life of a Fat Flusher

We are what we repeatedly do. Excellence, then, is not an act, but a habit.

—ARISTOTLE

The Fat Flush lifestyle involves much more than dietary changes. This exciting way of life is full of daily habits that encourage you to focus on yourself—and feel healthy and gorgeous. You'll have the energy and zest to live your life to the fullest each and every day! Dare I say some of these daily—and weekly—activities are true-blue indulgences, and not of the variety that are labeled "cheats." Here are my tried and true favorites, recognized by any Fat Flusher as notable reasons why the Fat Flush lifestyle, though low on sugar, is absolutely sweet.

OIL PULLING

To keep a lamp burning, we have to keep putting oil in it.

—MOTHER TERESA

Oil pulling is a simple yet highly beneficial method of cleansing your mouth as well as detoxing your entire system. Your mouth is the repository of a tremendous amount of bacteria that can impact different areas of your body. Dentists who practice holistic and biological dentistry believe that each tooth is connected to an organ. If that tooth has a root canal (even under a crown that x-rays don't pick up), is an implant, or even has been pulled, leaving behind a cavitation (hole in the jawbone), you can experience a whole host of health challenges in the associated meridian line of that tooth. This means that your unresolved digestive problem (teeth 2, 3, 28, and 29), irritable bowel syndrome (tooth 6), or even liver dysfunction (teeth 11 and 12) may be associated with the anaerobic bacteria seeping into your system from root canals, implants, and cavitations affecting those teeth. This can dramatically impact your system, making you ill in varying degrees.

To perform oil pulling, simply use two tablespoons of a healthy oil (my favorites are unrefined coconut oil, extra virgin olive oil, and untoasted sesame oil) and swish it vigorously around in your mouth for about 20 minutes. If you don't have time to complete the full 20 minutes, keep in mind that as long as you keep the oil in your mouth for at least 3 minutes, you will get major benefits. Aim to oil-pull first thing in the morning before you get out of bed, because when you get up and move around, the body cools down and sequesters the mobilized toxins from the night back into your tissues. I like to keep the oil in a cup on my nightstand to accomplish this task with ease. Oil pulling is such an inexpensive yet powerful method to cleanse toxins!

DRY BRUSHING

Doctors pour drugs of which they know little, to cure diseases of which they know less, into human beings of whom they know nothing.
—VOLTAIRE

Another technique that should become a ritual is one that stimulates lymphatic flow: dry-brush massage or skin brushing. Dry-brush massage promotes lymph flow and blood circulation, stimulates oil-producing glands in your skin, and helps enhance your immune system. As you may remember, your lympth system is your body's garbage collector. Doing this simple technique will help move out toxins while helping to lessen the appearance of cellulite; rebuild new, strong connective tissue; and promote toned, supple skin, especially as you lose weight.

Your skin is the largest organ of your body, and dry brushing is one of the best things you can do for it. Your skin is designed to help rid your body of wastes as you perspire. Dry brushing will remove dead layers of skin, open the pores, and remove toxins, leaving a youthful, healthy glow.

To get started, find a good brush at your local bath and beauty store, health food store, or department store. Look for a medium-firm brush with natural bristles—nylon or other synthetic bristles tend to be sharp and might damage your skin. Select a brush at least as large as the palm of your hand, with a long handle to reach your back.

Keep your brush clean by washing it frequently in warm, soapy water. Make sure it air-dries completely before you use it again. Once a week, soak your brush for 30 minutes in a solution of one quart of water and a few drops of Clorox bleach or tea tree oil (a natural disinfectant).

In case you were wondering why we waited until phase 2 to introduce the Fat Flush dry-brush massage, it's because most people who start the Fat Flush Plan have weakened connective tissues from years of sluggish lymph flow and accumulated toxins. Dry brushing this damaged tissue can cause bruising and discomfort. By phase 2, though, your connective tissues should be stronger and more resilient, and dry brushing will be very therapeutic.

You can dry-brush yourself at any time, but we don't advise waiting until the last few minutes before bedtime, as the brushing tends to have a stimulating effect that might interfere with sleep. If you dry-brush first thing in the morning, you'll feel energized all day. You'll probably want to shower or bathe after brushing, to wash away the dead skin.

The Fat Flush Dry-Brush Massage—Five Minutes, Two Times a Week

Feel free to work your way up to five times a week. Your skin will thank you for it, and so will your lymphatic system.

1. Open the primary lymphatic ducts by gently finger-massaging just below your collarbone and on the left and right groin areas. This only takes a few seconds.
2. Begin the brush massage with the soles of your feet. Brush vigorously in a circular motion. How firmly you press depends on how toned and healthy your skin is. As your skin becomes healthier, you will be able to apply more pressure, create better circulation, and bring increased energy into the skin. Using short, upward strokes, gradually move over your feet and legs. Continue brushing upward over your stomach to your breasts and over your buttocks to your waist.
3. Repeat the circular motion on the palms of your hands and then use short, upward strokes on your hands and arms. Brush down from your neck out to your shoulders and down to your breasts and down your back. As with other massage techniques, always stroke toward your heart.

Don't brush skin that's irritated or bruised. And avoid brushing your face—the skin is too sensitive there.

GROUNDING

We often forget that we are nature. Nature is not something separate from us. So when we say that we have lost our connection to nature, we have lost our connection to ourselves.

—ANDY GOLDSWORTHY

Grounding, or connecting daily to the earth, is an effortless form of releasing static electricity and neutralizing free radicals. Why? Science has proved that the earth is teeming with negatively charged electrons. A detachment from these electrons can cause a multitude of problems, including restless nights that lead to lethargic days, seemingly ceaseless stress (along with stress eating), and inflammation—the culprit in chronic health problems from obesity to cardiovascular disease to cancer.

How?

When connected to the earth, these electrons—nature's most abundant source of anti-inflammatories—act as antioxidants and instantaneously begin to neutralize the positively charged free radicals that create inflammation, stress, and disease.

Fluctuating cortisol levels are a key reason behind poor sleep. A lack of sleep then increases the stress hormone, stimulating hunger, which interferes with the body's ability to break down carbohydrates properly, thereby leading to sleep-deprived weight gain. But when you're regularly grounded, your body has assistance to stabilize your cortisol levels.

In fact, researchers in a groundbreaking study in the *Journal of Complementary and Alternative Medicine* wrote that "grounding the human body to earth ('earthing') during sleep reduces night-time levels of cortisol and resynchronizes cortisol hormone secretion more in alignment with the natural 24-hour circadian rhythm pattern."

When we feel like we need to clear our minds and recenter ourselves, you might think of metaphoric phrases like "getting back to our roots," or "coming back down to earth." In this case, it's much more literal.

While it's highly recommended for your well-being to get outside and take in nature, even a beautiful hike won't necessarily give you a good dose of "vitamin G" because we no longer walk barefoot or wear hides on our feet. Leather-soled shoes that permit the conduction of the earth's natural electrons are becoming more and more a thing of the past, and they have been replaced with synthetic plastic or rubber soles.

So while a stroll out in nature is good for the soul, it won't give you the same healing qualities that placing your bare feet on a plush spread of grass does. But what about those hot summer days (or overly chilly summer nights) that coax us inside? And although it's a nice idea, we certainly can't sleep under the stars every night. So how do we connect?

The good news is, we can now experience the earth's healing energy just as easily and safely indoors with Earthing technology. Discovered by Clint Ober, a pioneer in the cable TV industry, it's one of the most brilliant technological discoveries of the twenty-first century.

Earthing products are made from conductive fabric and materials—the fitted sheets, half sheets, universal mat, and wrist and ankle bands easily attach to an included ground cord that you can insert directly into the ground port of any electrical wall outlet or connect to an optional ground rod if your home or office does not have ground wall outlets. These products make it easy to ground yourself indoors while sleeping, working, or playing (and it only takes about three seconds of setup time!).

Do visit the Earthing section of Uni Key's website at http://www.unikeyhealth.com/earthing and Earthing's official website at https://www.earthing.com to bring grounding into your home today.

As for me, I enjoy sound sleep each night nestled on my Earthing fitted sheet and can truly attest to the positive impact of vitamin G.

AROMATHERAPY BATHS

I have learned, as a rule of thumb, never to ask whether you can do something. Say, instead, that you are doing it. Then fasten your seat belt. The most remarkable things follow.

—JULIA CAMERON

I am a huge proponent of relaxing, therapeutic bathing. Hot baths are an excellent way to reduce stress, soothe muscles, care for skin, and encourage detox by opening the pores and stimulating lymph flow—releasing toxins through perspiration.

Adding essential oils to your bath takes an already relaxing and health-promoting ritual to the next level. Essential oils are distilled from the flowers, leaves, and roots of wild or organically grown plants. The oils are quickly absorbed into your body through the skin or are inhaled through your nose, and they send a soothing message to the brain, initiating feelings of well-being and harmony. These stress busters can reduce cortisol levels, decrease fat deposits and water retention, improve muscle soreness, and increase beneficial sleep. If Fat Flush had a smell, it would be the aroma of essential oils.

They've been credited with numerous effects, including:

• Reducing water retention and fat deposits
• Alleviating stress and anxiety—which reduces cortisol, which in turn aids weight loss
• Reducing muscle soreness

Studies have also shown that certain essential oils can stimulate the hypothalamus to:

• **Suppress your appetite.** Alan Hirsch, MD, director of the Smell and Taste Research Foundation in Chicago, has shown that peppermint activates the portion of the hypothalamus that regulates our sense of fullness.
• **Relieve pain.** Studies in England and elsewhere have noted the powerful effect of lavender and rose oils to overcome intense pain.

Through the hypothalamus, their scents inspire the thalamus gland to produce encephalin, a natural painkiller and antidepressant.
• **Stimulate your immune and lymphatic systems.** Lemon and other oils trigger the release of noradrenaline, which both fights fatigue and boosts your immune and lymph systems.

Plus, let's face it—they just smell good! The pungent scent of cinnamon, the spicy aroma of bergamot, the zesty smells of lemon and orange stimulate your senses and reawaken your awareness of your physical self. There are many utilitarian reasons to lose weight and become fit—combating heart disease, lengthening your life span, boosting your energy levels. But it's nice to remember that the ultimate purpose of these plans is to enable you to enjoy your life, take pleasure in your body, and renew your spirit.

So open up to aromatherapy by putting some essential oils into your warm bath, enabling the oils to penetrate your skin. Choose two or more oils from the lymph-friendly essential oils list below, and add a total of 2–5 drops dispersed into the flowing water as you fill your tub. (Don't overdo it—these are potent substances, and using them to excess could produce an allergic reaction or other unwelcome side effects.) Then soak for 20 minutes—at the end of the afternoon, to help you release workday stress and transition to a relaxing evening, or an hour or so before bedtime to help you sleep.

For Fat Flushers, the following oils provide the healthiest and most beautifying benefits:

• **Rose.** Rose oil acts as an antidepressant and anti-inflammatory that improves circulation and can help reduce heart palpitations, cravings, and stress.
• **Lavender.** Lavender can also reduce cravings, stress, and inflammation, as well as fight fungal infections, improve skin disorders (including acne, psoriasis, eczema, and wrinkles), lower blood pressure, and aid in digestion by stimulating production of bile and gastric juices.
• **Sandalwood.** Sandalwood oil relaxes the adrenal glands, which are so often fatigued, effectively lowering stress and encouraging deeper sleep.
• **Thyme.** Thyme oil builds immunity, fights pathogenic bacteria, stimulates the lymphatics, reduces inflammation, and is antiparasitic.
• **Geranium.** Geranium oil supports adrenal function and works as an antibacterial, antifungal, antitumor, and anti-inflammatory agent.
• **Marjoram.** Marjoram oil has a calming effect that reduces stress and can improve diabetes, irritable bowel syndrome, rheumatism, fatigue, and muscle tension.

- **Cedarwood.** Cedarwood oil fortifies and strengthens lungs and promotes quality sleep.
- **Rosemary.** Rosemary oil is especially regenerating, restorative, and detoxifying, relieving pain, stress, and indigestion.
- **Lemon.** Lemon oil improves clarity and disinfects your system; you can even use a few drops in water for a homemade household cleaning spray.
- **Juniper.** Juniper oil promotes toxic waste elimination with its laxative properties. It also reduces fluid retention and helps cleanse the emotions, calming an anxious mind.
- **Lemongrass.** Lemongrass oil tones and strengthens connective tissues, stimulates lymphatic tissues, and purges excess fluid from your system.
- **Grapefruit.** Grapefruit oil is an antimicrobial that helps dissolve fatty deposits and promotes toning and tightening of your body.
- **Peppermint.** Peppermint oil alleviates flatulence, bloating, and upset stomach.
- **Chamomile.** Chamomile is the ultimate calming oil and is often helpful in promoting sleep.

It is important to check the label when purchasing essential oils. The label should state that the oils have been analyzed by a gas chromatograph–mass spectrometer to ensure safety and effectiveness. This is really the only way to know that they are high quality and do not include any petrochemicals, fractions of cheaper oils, synthetic fragrance, or other degrading chemicals.

If you want the benefits of essential oils but do not have a bathtub to use them in, you can put a few drops of the oils on cold lightbulbs in lamps. The heat of the lightbulb when it is turned on will diffuse the scent. You can also purchase an oil diffuser or apply the oil directly to your skin. For skin application, apply at the pulse points and on the bottom of your feet, which is, surprisingly, the best location for absorption.

EPSOM SALT BATH

Be not afraid of going slowly, be afraid only of standing still.
—THEODORE ROOSEVELT

Epsom salt baths are a trusty home remedy with fantastic restorative abilities for your skin and muscles. This supersalt soak also has detoxifying properties that provide a number of supplemental benefits to Fat Flushers on their health-seeking journey. The Epsom salt itself is actually magnesium sulfate, and soaking in an Epsom salt bath is an excellent way to increase the magnesium levels in your body. The sulfate half of the magnesium sulfate pair has perks all its own, helping in the formation of brain tissue, joint protein, and the strength of the digestive tract's walls. These baths will leave your body feeling better with firmer skin, more relaxed muscles, and a fitter frame.

For your Epsom salt baths, add two cups of Epsom salt to a tub full of hot water and soak for 20 minutes.

CASTOR OIL PACKS

It is supposed to be a professional secret, but I'll tell you anyway. We doctors do nothing. We only help and encourage the doctor within.
—ALBERT SCHWEITZER

This is probably the least well known of the detox methods, but perhaps the most therapeutic of them all. Castor oil packs rock. They stimulate the liver and gallbladder, support the bile, and draw toxins out of the body. Castor oil normalizes liver enzymes, decreases elevated cholesterol levels, and provides a sense of well-being. I include castor oil treatments with bathing rituals because, like the other bathing methods, you are using a healing liquid to infuse your body through the skin.

Using castor oil packs is an easy and rewarding experience. All you need is a pack of 100 percent pure, cold-pressed castor oil; wool (not cotton) flannel; and a heating pad. To take your detoxification to the next level, follow these simple steps:

1. Fold the wool flannel into three or four layers and soak it with castor oil.
2. Place the soaked flannel in a baking dish and heat it slowly in the oven until it is hot to your touch.
3. Lie down, gently rub three tablespoons of castor oil on your abdomen, and then place the soaked flannel across your abdomen.
4. Cover the soaked flannel with a plastic wrap or plastic garbage bag.
5. Finally, cover the soaked flannel with the heating pad for one hour to keep it comfortably hot.

When you finish, wash the oil from your abdomen. You can keep the oil-soaked flannel sealed in a plastic wrap or place it in a plastic storage bag for further use, since castor oil does not become rancid as quickly as many other oils.

As a gentle detox, I recommend that you use the castor oil pack once a day for three days in a row, then take three days off, and then use it for another three consecutive days. Continue this pattern every week or every other week, depending upon your liver enzyme levels. If you suffer from frequent colds, infections, or chronic fatigue syndrome, consider using the castor oil pack on a daily basis for two weeks out of every month.

Daily, weekly, and monthly rituals will soon become second nature to your Fat Flush lifestyle. As Sarah Ban Breathnach so wisely observed, "Start thinking of yourself as an artist and your life as a work-in-progress. Works-in-progress are never perfect. But changes can be made. . . . Art evolves. So does life. Art is never stagnant. Neither is life. The beautiful, authentic life you are creating for yourself is your art. It's the highest art."

SELECTED FAT FLUSH SUPERSTAPLES

To be nobody but yourself in a world which is doing its best, night and day, to make you everybody else means to fight the hardest battle which any human being can fight.

—E. E. Cummings

Cranberries

Of course cranberries are on this list. These ruby-red jewels are chock-full of important antioxidants, vitamins, and organic acids. Among the most potent elements in cranberries are polyphenols, a kind of plant-based antioxidant that has powerful health-inducing effects. Just 2 ounces of fresh cranberries contain 373 milligrams of polyphenols, more than much larger servings of oranges, broccoli, blueberries, or strawberries. These brilliant berries are also vital aids to liver detox because they contain exceedingly high levels of lifesaving antioxidants that provide crucial support during detox protocols.

The weight loss benefits of cranberry come from its ability to kick the lymphatic system into gear. When the lymph isn't flowing properly, excess fluid that isn't draining from our tissues causes them to swell. These bloated, inflamed tissues can add up to 10 or 15 pounds to your weight and cause you to swell two extra sizes. Specifically talking cellulite, the proanthocyanidins in cranberry strengthen connective tissue by blocking the destructive activity of certain enzymes.

I recommend faithfully drinking eight glasses of cran-water throughout each day. It's also a taste treat to add cran-water to your smoothies, which offsets the sweetness from fruit.

To prepare, simply mix one ounce of 100 percent unsweetened cranberry juice with seven ounces of water. Multiply the recipe as needed to have enough for your eight daily glasses easily on hand.

Flax Seeds

These classic seeds are loaded with fiber, which keeps toxins moving out of your body—where they should be. Flax seeds have also been found to power up the immune system and even be an effective cancer fighter. They can be of particular benefit to postmenopausal women because the lignans in the fibrous shell counteract the cell-proliferating power of excess estrogen.

From flaxseed crackers to an excellent smoothie add-in, there are many ways to work flax's healthful crunch into your routine.

Chia Seeds

This ancient superfood packs a real punch. Extremely nutrient dense, one small seed contains nearly fifty energizing nutrients. They are gluten-free and abundant in vitamin C, protein, minerals, vegetable-based calcium, essential fatty acids, and fiber.

You can sprinkle them on salads or add them to a smoothie without altering the taste.

Dandelion Root

Loaded with nutrients and minerals, it's powerful for stimulating liver function and detox. One such nutrient is inulin, a fiber-like substance that functions as a prebiotic to help nourish the friendly bacteria in the gut. The humble dandelion root is also good for lowering blood sugar and boosting the overall health of the microbiome.

It's the perfect swap or trade-off to have in place of coffee for those of you on a detox. Another easy and delicious option is to add it to your daily smoothie.

Beets

Full of betaine, beets are a prominent protector of the liver against the damaging effects of alcohol. Betaine also thins the bile and helps it move freely within the bile ducts, and it is an incredibly rich dietary source of nitric oxide and antioxidants.

Beets tend to have a bad reputation when it comes to taste, but I find them to be quite delicious when grated and sprinkled over a salad.

Seaweed Gomasio

A healthy alternative to plain table salt, this traditional sesame salt has been used for centuries in Asia. It's made from organically grown sesame seeds roasted and ground with sea salt and three sea vegetables—dulse, nori, and kombu, all of which are rich in trace minerals. As a source of high-quality protein, calcium, iron, iodine, and a superior range of amino acids—including methionine, tryptophan, and lysine—seaweed gomasio provides nutrients that are often missing in vegetable protein sources. Sea vegetables, due to their sodium alginate content, are also well known to be protective against environmental pollutants.

Try it on salads, vegetables, popcorn, and corn on the cob in place of salt. It also heightens flavor in salad dressings and marinades.

Cumin

Found in seed or ground form in Middle Eastern, East Indian, African, and Mexican cuisines, cumin is a surprising weight loss aid that also relieves gas, colic, and digestive-connected headaches. A powerful free-radical scavenger, cumin also improves liver function and enhances the primo detox antioxidant, glutathione.

It's a great addition to wake up beans (especially red beans), dips, marinades, stews, lamb, beef, and other spice mixtures.

My Fat Flush Shopping List

The important things in life cannot be gotten in advance.
They must be gathered fresh every day.

—GEORGE REGAS

Many of the foods on the shopping list can be purchased at your local health food store or farmer's market; whereas others are available in supermarkets. Naturally, non-GMO organic produce (vegetables and fruit) is preferable (not only are these veggies and fruits tastier and fresher, but they do not have all those nasty pesticides, fungicides, and heavy metals your liver has to break down). For this reason, I am providing the names of some of the easier-to-obtain brands in parentheses. But please check even the brand names list yourself because formulations and therefore ingredients can change periodically.

Also note that while in the grocery store, it's important to pay special attention to the following 11 foods, which are especially likely to contain GMOs. Purchase organic only!

- Corn (as in corn oil, cornmeal, cornstarch, corn syrup, hominy, polenta, and other corn-based ingredients)
- Canola (as in canola oil)
- Cottonseed (as in cottonseed oil)
- Sugar beets (as in "sugar" in an ingredient, which is almost certainly a combination of sugar from both sugar cane and GM sugar beets)
- Soybeans (as in soybean oil, soy protein, soy lecithin, soy milk, tofu, and other soy-based ingredients)
- Alfalfa
- Apples, all varieties
- Papaya (from Hawaii and China)
- Potatoes
- Yellow squash and zucchini (look for those labeled organic or grown from non-GMO seed)

Let's start shopping!

PHASE 1: THE TWO-WEEK FAT FLUSH

Eggs

- Omega-3–enriched (The Happy Egg Co., Vital Farms, Organic Valley, The Country Hen, and Pilgrim's Pride EggsPlus)

Protein: Fish

Fresh

- Bass
- Cod
- Grouper
- Haddock
- Halibut
- Mackerel
- Mahi-mahi
- Orange roughy
- Perch
- Pike
- Pollock
- Salmon
- Sardines
- Snapper
- Sole
- Squid
- Trout
- Tuna
- Whitefish

Canned

- Crabmeat (Wild Planet, Vital Choice Seafood, Crown Prince, Skip Jack Tuna, Bar Harbor)
- Mackerel
- Salmon
- Sardines
- Tuna

Protein: Shellfish

- Calamari
- Crab

* Lobster
* Scallops
* Shrimp

Protein: Poultry

* White meat of skinned turkey and chicken, either fresh, frozen, or ground (preferably free range and hormone-free, such as Tecumseh Farms Organic, Mary's Chicken, Good Earth Farms, and local farms)

Protein: Meats

Beef

Preferably grass fed, such as Aspen Ridge, Ayrshire Farm, Holy Cow, and local farms.

* Brisket
* Chuck
* Eye of round
* Flank
* London broil
* Round
* Rump
* Sirloin

Lamb

* Leg
* Loin
* Rib

Veal

* Loin
* Rib
* Shoulder

Other Meats

* Elk
* Bison (buffalo)
* Ostrich
* Venison

Vegetables

- Alfalfa sprouts
- Artichoke hearts
- Arugula
- Asparagus
- Bell peppers, red, green, and orange
- Bamboo shoots
- Broccoli
- Brussels sprouts
- Burdock
- Cabbage
- Carrots
- Cauliflower
- Celery
- Chinese cabbage
- Chives
- Collard greens
- Cucumbers
- Daikon
- Eggplant
- Endive
- Escarole
- Green beans
- Hearts of palm
- Jicama
- Kale
- Loose-leaf lettuce, red or green
- Mung bean sprouts
- Mushrooms
- Mustard greens
- Okra
- Olives
- Onions
- Parsley
- Radicchio
- Radishes
- Rhubarb
- Romaine lettuce
- Sea vegetables such as agar-agar, hijiki, kombu, nori, or wakame or a sea veggie–based seasoning (like Eden Seaweed Gomasio, kelp granules, or dulse flakes from Maine)
- Snow peas
- Spaghetti squash

- Spinach
- Tomatillos
- Tomatoes
- Tomato products: Mom's tomato sauces are my favorite (momspastasauce.com). Also, you can find more tomato products on ThriveMarket.com like Jovial, Bionaturae.
- Water chestnuts
- Watercress
- Yellow squash
- Zucchini

Fruits

Fresh, frozen, or canned in natural unsweetened juices and drained. Frozen brands include Cascadian Farms and Stahlbush Island Farms.

- Apples
- Avocados
- Berries (blueberries, blackberries, and raspberries)
- Cherries
- Cranberries (available seasonally)
- Grapefruit
- Lemons. Fresh is best, although Santa Cruz Organic 100% Lemon Juice Not from Concentrate will do.
- Limes. Fresh is best, although Santa Cruz Organic 100% Lime Juice Not from Concentrate will do.
- Nectarines
- Oranges
- Peaches
- Pears
- Plums
- Pomegranates (available seasonally)
- Strawberries

Herbs, Spices, and All Accompaniments

Look for non-GMO and nonirradiated varieties from Frontier Herbs and The Spice Hunter.

- Anise
- Apple cider vinegar (Bragg's organic apple cider vinegar is the best!)
- Bay leaves
- Cayenne

- Chia seeds, whole organic or chemical-free chia seeds in bulk. You do not need to grind chia seeds to derive the benefits (Spectrum, Uni Key chia seeds).
- Cinnamon
- Cloves
- Coconut vinegar (Tropical Traditions)
- Coriander
- Cream of tartar
- Cumin
- Dill (fresh or dried)
- Dried mustard
- Fennel (fresh or ground)
- Flax seeds, organic whole brown or golden-yellow flax seeds in bulk to be ground daily as needed in a coffee grinder, blender, or food processor on the fine setting (Omega)
- Garlic (fresh or garlic powder)
- Ginger (fresh or dried)
- Hemp seeds. You can buy hemp seed in bulk to be ground daily as needed in a coffee grinder, blender, or food processor on the fine setting. You can also purchase shelled hemp seed if you do not want to buy your own (Nutiva).
- Onion powder
- Turmeric

Oils and Sprays
- Avocado oil spray (such as Chosen Foods)
- Coconut oil (such as Nutiva and Tropical Traditions)
- High-lignan and regular flaxseed oil (such as Omega and Barleans)
- Flavored fish oil (such as Carlson's), for those who cannot tolerate flaxseed oil
- MCT (medium-chain triglyceride) oil (such as Now, Nature's Way, Jarrow)

Bone Broths
- Beef, chicken, fish, vegetable broth (Pacific Foods). I especially encourage purchasing ready-made bone broth, as it is heavily featured in the Fat Flush recipes (Wise Choice Market, Kettle & Fire, Pacific Foods, LonoLife, The Osso Good Co., Au Bon Broth, Bondafide Provisions).

Juices and Other Drinks

- Cranberry juice, unsweetened (Knudsen's, Trader Joe's, Mountain Sun)
- Dandelion root tea, coffee
- Fennel, ginger, and peppermint tea
- Organic fair-trade coffee

Protein Sources

- Pea and rice protein powders that are low carb, non-GMO, unsweetened, and organic and, if possible, with third-party testing for heavy metals (Pea & Rice Fat Flush Body Protein and Body Ecology Fermented Plant Protein)
- Tempeh
- Tofu (Mori-Nu, White Wave)
- Whey (nonvegan) protein powders that are hormone-free, unheated, nondenatured, lactose-free, free of added sugars or artificial sweeteners like aspartame, sucralose, or Splenda, with about 20 grams of protein per serving and negligible carbohydrates from nonmutated A2 milk (Fat Flush Whey and Designs for Health Whey)

Sweeteners

- Flora-Key, stevia (SweetLeaf Stevia), monk fruit and erythritol (Lakanto)

Friendly Carbohydrates

- Shirataki noodles—made from glucomannan (a type of gummy fiber)

PHASE 2: THE METABOLIC RESET

You may have these foods in addition to the ones on the phase 1 list.

Friendly Carbs

- Quinoa
- Steel-cut or rolled oats

Vegetables

- Beets
- Butternut and acorn squash
- Green peas, fresh or frozen
- Sweet potato

Fruits

- Bananas
- Pineapple

PHASE 3: LIFESTYLE EATING PLAN

You may have these foods in addition to the ones on the phase 1 and phase 2 lists.

Dairy Products

Companies such as Nancy's and Horizon offer a wide variety of organic dairy products.

- Buttermilk (prepared using milk from Horizon, Organic Valley, local farm)
- Cheddar cheese
- Cottage cheese, full fat (Friendship, Old Home)
- Cream
- Cream cheese
- Goat cheese
- Grated Parmesan cheese (occasionally)
- Ghee (Organic Valley, Purity Farms, Pure Indian Foods)
- Mozzarella cheese
- Parmesan cheese
- Ricotta cheese (Calabro)
- Romano cheese
- Sour cream
- String cheese
- Sweet butter
- Swiss cheese
- Yogurt, plain Greek full fat

   Make sure all dairy products are full fat and, as much as possible, are from organically raised, grass-fed cows. If intolerant to dairy, use coconut or almond substitutes like coconut cream, full-fat coconut milk (Trader Joe's), and almond milk (Natural Directions).

Protein: Poultry

Turkey

• Organic, nitrate-free turkey bacon (Apple Farms), turkey jerky (Perky Jerky, Krave Jerky, Golden Valley, New Primal)

Protein: Meat

Beef

• Beef jerky (Epic, B.U.L.K., New Primal, Paleo Snacks)

Friendly Carbs

• Rutabaga
• Turnips

Starchy Vegetables

• Baked potato
• Corn on the cob
• Pumpkin
• Red potatoes

Beans

• Adzuki beans
• Black beans
• Chickpeas
• Kidney beans
• Pinto beans

Canned beans are fine if you rinse and drain them.

Cereals and Grains

Gluten-free and non-GMO.

• Lentil and quinoa pasta (Ancient Grain)
• Brown rice
• Popcorn (Good Health Half Naked Organic Sea Salt Popcorn)

Crackers and Chips

Gluten-free and non-GMO.

- Brown flax or rice crackers (Mary's Gone Crackers)
- Corn tortillas
- Dill, rosemary, tomato, and savory flax crackers (Doctor in the Kitchen)
- Organic golden flax crackers (Foods Alive)
- Seaweed snacks and seaweed chips (SeaSnax)
- Three-seed crackers (RW Garcia)

Gluten-Free and Flour Alternatives

- Almond flour
- Chickpea flour
- Coconut flour
- Paleo coconut wraps (The Pure Wraps)
- Raw wraps (Green Leaf Foods)
- Tapioca flour
- Tigernut flour (Organic Gemini)

Special Occasional Snacks, Treats, and Sweets

- Protein bars (Epic)
- Baked potato chips made with olive oil or avocado oil (Good Health Kettle Chips)
- Granola made with raw, unpasteurized honey and maple syrup (Prime Island, Platte Clove Naturals)

Fruits

- Cantaloupe
- Grapes
- Honeydew
- Kiwi
- Pineapple
- Watermelon

Special Occasion Fruit

- Dried fruit (Organic Traditions, Peeled Organic)

Nuts and Seeds

- Caraway seeds
- Chestnuts
- Filberts
- Macadamia nuts
- Peanuts
- Pecans
- Poppy seeds
- Pumpkin seeds
- Raw almonds
- Sunflower seeds
- Tigernuts (Organic Gemini, Supreme Peeled)
- Walnuts

This category also includes peanut, almond, and sesame butters and tahini (Kevala, Living Intentions). Be sure that all nut and seed butters are free of canola, sunflower, soybean, corn, and safflower oil and that they only contain healthy oils, if at all.

Herbs, Spices, and All Accompaniments

- Basil
- Chinese five-spice powder
- Chipotle powder (Simply Organic Chipotle Powder, Out of Mexico Chipotle Powder)
- Dijon mustard
- Oregano
- Paprika:
  - Hungarian paprika (Bascom's Hungarian Paprika Spices, Szeged Hot Paprika Powder)
  - Smoked paprika (Simply Organic Smoked Paprika, Chiquilin Smoked Paprika)
- Rosemary
- Sage
- Sea salt such as Selina Naturally Celtic Sea Salt. (If on a sodium-restricted diet, choose Makai Pure Deep Sea Salt, which has the highest potassium level of any comparable sea salt on the market.)
- Tarragon
- Thyme

Condiments

- Angostura bitters
- Avocado mayonnaise (Primal Kitchen, Chosen Foods, Thrive Market)
- Capers

Special Occasion

- Gluten-free tamari (San-J)
- Umeboshi paste (Eden, Ohsawa)

Cooking Products and Extras

- Carob powder
- Cocoa powder

Flavor Extracts

- Organic vanilla, almond, and other assorted extracts (Simply Organic, Olive Nation, Nature's Flavors)

Oils and Sprays

- Avocado oil (Spectrum Naturals, Primal Kitchen, La Tourangelle)
- Extra virgin and unfiltered olive oils (California Estates, Lucini, Napa Valley Naturals, Bragg)
- Macadamia oil (Piping Rock Health Products, Mac Nut Oil, Roland)
- Sesame and toasted sesame oil (Spectrum, La Tourangelle, Trader Joe's)
- Olive oil sprays (Spectrum Naturals, Lucini, Napa Valley Naturals)

Bonus Foods

- Shredded coconut (Let's Do Organic, Bob's Red Mill, Anthony's Goods)
- Full-fat unsweetened coconut milk and almond milk (Silk, SO Delicious, Native Forest, Pacific Foods, Tropical Traditions)
- Sour cream and cream cheese (365 Whole Foods, Horizon, Organic Valley, Nancy's)

Baking Powder

- Aluminum-free brands (Royal, Rumford, Price, McCormick's)
- Low-sodium, cereal-free brands (Cellu, Featherweight)

Thickeners

- Arrowroot
- Kuzu

Juices and Other Drinks

- Low-sodium vegetable juices (Low Sodium V-8 Juice, Muir Glen Tomato Juice, Muir Glen 100% Vegetable Juice, and Knudsen Organic Very Veggie Juice)

Acceptable Teas and Coffees

- Fair-trade and organic dandelion root and red tea (rooibos tea)
- Organic coffee
- Fennel tea
- Ginger tea
- Peppermint tea

Special Occasion Alcohol

- Organic and sulfite-free (Coturri Winery, Frey, Fetzer, Organic Wine Company, HoneyRun Winery, Hallcrest Vineyards, Marcel Lapierre, Stellar Organics, Spartico No Sulfur Added, China Bend Vineyards, Trader Joe's)

Sweeteners

- Yacon syrup (Organic Traditions, Sunfood Superfoods, Therapeutic Laboratories, Swanson Health)

Part Two

My Fat Flush Journal

PREPARING FOR WEEK 1

If we wait until we're ready, we'll be waiting for the rest of our lives.

—LEMONY SNICKET

TODAY'S DATE _____

MY PHASE _____ GOAL _____

_____

MEASUREMENTS

- Bust/Chest _____
- Waist _____
- Hips _____
- Thighs _____
- Weight _____

HOW REACHING MY GOAL WILL CHANGE MY LIFE

_____

_____

_____

_____

_____

_____

_____

THE BIGGEST CHALLENGES I ANTICIPATE THIS WEEK

_____

_____

_____

_____

_____

_____

A HABIT TAKES 21 DAYS TO FORM. MY HEALTHY HABIT (PHYSICAL OR SPRITIUAL) I'M BEGINNING OR CONTINUING TO DEVELOP THIS WEEK

_____

_____

_____

_____

_____

_____

MY MANTRA FOR THE WEEK

_____

_____

_____

_____

_____

_____

_____

WEEK 1: DAY 1

Life is not against me. Life is absolutely on my side.
—*Michael Bernard Beckwith*

TODAY'S DATE _____

MEALS, BEVERAGES, SNACKS, AND SUPPLEMENTS

• Upon rising _____

• Before breakfast _____

• Breakfast _____

_____

• Midmorning snack _____

• Before lunch _____

• Lunch _____

_____

_____

_____

• 4 P.M. snack_____

• Before dinner_____

• Dinner_____

_____

_____

_____

• Midevening _____

HOURS SLEPT LAST NIGHT AND QUALITY OF SLEEP _____

_____

_____

_____

_____

EXERCISE _____

_____

_____

_____

HOW I IMPROVED FROM YESTERDAY _____

_____

_____

_____

_____

HOW I FEEL PHYSICALLY _____

_____

_____

_____

HOW I FEEL MENTALLY_____

_____

_____

_____

HOW I OVERCAME A CHALLENGE _____

_____

_____

_____

WHAT I FEEL GRATEFUL FOR TODAY _____

_____

_____

_____

_____

_____

WEEK 1: DAY 2

Doubt kills more dreams than failure ever will.
— *Karim Seddiki*

TODAY'S DATE _____

MEALS, BEVERAGES, SNACKS, AND SUPPLEMENTS

- Upon rising _____
- Before breakfast _____
- Breakfast _____
  _____
- Midmorning snack _____
- Before lunch _____
- Lunch _____
  _____
  _____
  _____
- 4 P.M. snack_____
- Before dinner_____
- Dinner_____
  _____
  _____
  _____
- Midevening _____

HOURS SLEPT LAST NIGHT AND QUALITY OF SLEEP _____
_____
_____
_____
_____

EXERCISE _____

_____

_____

_____

HOW I IMPROVED FROM YESTERDAY _____

_____

_____

_____

_____

HOW I FEEL PHYSICALLY _____

_____

_____

_____

_____

HOW I FEEL MENTALLY_____

_____

_____

_____

HOW I OVERCAME A CHALLENGE _____

_____

_____

_____

_____

WHAT I FEEL GRATEFUL FOR TODAY _____

_____

_____

_____

_____

_____

WEEK 1: DAY 3

> *Life is either a daring adventure or nothing.*
>
> —Helen Keller

TODAY'S DATE _____

MEALS, BEVERAGES, SNACKS, AND SUPPLEMENTS

• Upon rising _____

• Before breakfast _____

• Breakfast _____

_____

• Midmorning snack _____

• Before lunch _____

• Lunch _____

_____

_____

_____

• 4 P.M. snack_____

• Before dinner_____

• Dinner_____

_____

_____

_____

• Midevening _____

HOURS SLEPT LAST NIGHT AND QUALITY OF SLEEP _____

_____

_____

_____

_____

EXERCISE _____

_____

_____

_____

HOW I IMPROVED FROM YESTERDAY _____

_____

_____

_____

_____

HOW I FEEL PHYSICALLY _____

_____

_____

_____

_____

HOW I FEEL MENTALLY _____

_____

_____

_____

HOW I OVERCAME A CHALLENGE _____

_____

_____

_____

_____

WHAT I FEEL GRATEFUL FOR TODAY _____

_____

_____

_____

_____

_____

WEEK 1: DAY 4

If you stumble, make it part of the dance.

—*Anonymous*

TODAY'S DATE _____

MEALS, BEVERAGES, SNACKS, AND SUPPLEMENTS

• Upon rising _____

• Before breakfast _____

• Breakfast _____

_____

• Midmorning snack _____

• Before lunch _____

• Lunch _____

_____

_____

_____

• 4 P.M. snack_____

• Before dinner_____

• Dinner_____

_____

_____

_____

• Midevening _____

HOURS SLEPT LAST NIGHT AND QUALITY OF SLEEP _____

_____

_____

_____

_____

EXERCISE _____

_____

_____

_____

HOW I IMPROVED FROM YESTERDAY _____

_____

_____

_____

_____

HOW I FEEL PHYSICALLY _____

_____

_____

_____

_____

HOW I FEEL MENTALLY_____

_____

_____

_____

HOW I OVERCAME A CHALLENGE _____

_____

_____

_____

_____

WHAT I FEEL GRATEFUL FOR TODAY _____

_____

_____

_____

_____

WEEK 1: DAY 5

> *You can't start the next chapter of your life if you keep re-reading the last one.*
>
> —*Lewis Carroll*

TODAY'S DATE _____

MEALS, BEVERAGES, SNACKS, AND SUPPLEMENTS

• Upon rising _____

• Before breakfast _____

• Breakfast _____

_____

• Midmorning snack _____

• Before lunch _____

• Lunch _____

_____

_____

_____

• 4 P.M. snack_____

• Before dinner_____

• Dinner_____

_____

_____

_____

• Midevening _____

HOURS SLEPT LAST NIGHT AND QUALITY OF SLEEP _____

_____

_____

_____

_____

EXERCISE _____

_____

_____

_____

HOW I IMPROVED FROM YESTERDAY _____

_____

_____

_____

_____

HOW I FEEL PHYSICALLY _____

_____

_____

_____

_____

HOW I FEEL MENTALLY_____

_____

_____

_____

HOW I OVERCAME A CHALLENGE _____

_____

_____

_____

_____

WHAT I FEEL GRATEFUL FOR TODAY _____

_____

_____

_____

_____

WEEK 1: DAY 6

We are all broken. That's how the light gets in.

—Ernest Hemingway

TODAY'S DATE _____

MEALS, BEVERAGES, SNACKS, AND SUPPLEMENTS

• Upon rising _____

• Before breakfast _____

• Breakfast _____

_____

• Midmorning snack _____

• Before lunch _____

• Lunch _____

_____

_____

_____

• 4 P.M. snack_____

• Before dinner_____

• Dinner_____

_____

_____

_____

• Midevening _____

HOURS SLEPT LAST NIGHT AND QUALITY OF SLEEP _____

_____

_____

_____

_____

EXERCISE _____

_____

_____

_____

HOW I IMPROVED FROM YESTERDAY _____

_____

_____

_____

_____

HOW I FEEL PHYSICALLY _____

_____

_____

_____

_____

HOW I FEEL MENTALLY_____

_____

_____

_____

HOW I OVERCAME A CHALLENGE _____

_____

_____

_____

_____

WHAT I FEEL GRATEFUL FOR TODAY _____

_____

_____

_____

_____

WEEK 1: DAY 7

> *There are only two ways to live your life. One is as though nothing is a miracle. The other is as though everything is.*
>
> —*Albert Einstein*

TODAY'S DATE _____

MEALS, BEVERAGES, SNACKS, AND SUPPLEMENTS

• Upon rising _____

• Before breakfast _____

• Breakfast _____

_____

• Midmorning snack _____

• Before lunch _____

• Lunch _____

_____

_____

_____

• 4 P.M. snack_____

• Before dinner_____

• Dinner_____

_____

_____

_____

• Midevening _____

HOURS SLEPT LAST NIGHT AND QUALITY OF SLEEP _____

_____

_____

_____

_____

Day 7

EXERCISE _____

_____

_____

_____

HOW I IMPROVED FROM YESTERDAY _____

_____

_____

_____

_____

HOW I FEEL PHYSICALLY _____

_____

_____

_____

_____

HOW I FEEL MENTALLY_____

_____

_____

_____

HOW I OVERCAME A CHALLENGE _____

_____

_____

_____

_____

WHAT I FEEL GRATEFUL FOR TODAY _____

_____

_____

_____

_____

_____

PREPARING FOR WEEK 2

You are never too old to set another goal or dream another dream.

—C. S. LEWIS

TODAY'S DATE _____

MY PHASE _____ GOAL _____

_____

MEASUREMENTS

- Bust/Chest _____
- Waist _____
- Hips _____
- Thighs _____
- Weight _____

OVER THE PAST WEEK, HERE'S WHAT I'VE NOTICED ABOUT:

- The fit of my clothes_____

  _____

- My sleep patterns _____

  _____

  _____

- My energy level_____

  _____

  _____

- My emotional well-being_____

  _____

  _____

- My skin_____

  _____

  _____

MY BIGGEST STRUGGLE

_____

_____

_____

_____

MY BEST COMPLIMENT

_____

_____

_____

_____

MY PROUDEST MOMENT

_____

_____

_____

_____

THE BIGGEST CHALLENGES I ANTICIPATE THIS WEEK

_____

_____

_____

_____

A HABIT TAKES 21 DAYS TO FORM. MY HEALTHY HABIT (PHYSICAL OR
SPRITIUAL) I'M BEGINNING OR CONTINUING TO DEVELOP THIS WEEK

_____

_____

_____

_____

_____

MY REWARD FOR A WEEK OF PROGRESS

_____

_____

_____

_____

_____

MY MANTRA FOR THE WEEK

_____

_____

_____

_____

REMINDER: HOW REACHING MY GOAL WILL CHANGE MY LIFE

_____

_____

_____

_____

WEEK 2: DAY 1

A strong woman looks a challenge dead in the eye and gives it a wink.

—*Gina Carey*

TODAY'S DATE _____

MEALS, BEVERAGES, SNACKS, AND SUPPLEMENTS

• Upon rising _____

• Before breakfast _____

• Breakfast _____

_____

• Midmorning snack _____

• Before lunch _____

• Lunch _____

_____

_____

_____

• 4 P.M. snack_____

• Before dinner_____

• Dinner_____

_____

_____

_____

• Midevening _____

HOURS SLEPT LAST NIGHT AND QUALITY OF SLEEP _____

_____

_____

_____

_____

EXERCISE _____

_____

_____

_____

HOW I IMPROVED FROM YESTERDAY _____

_____

_____

_____

_____

HOW I FEEL PHYSICALLY _____

_____

_____

_____

HOW I FEEL MENTALLY_____

_____

_____

_____

HOW I OVERCAME A CHALLENGE _____

_____

_____

_____

WHAT I FEEL GRATEFUL FOR TODAY _____

_____

_____

_____

_____

_____

WEEK 2: DAY 2

Life is like a coin. You can spend it any way you wish, but you only spend it once.

—Lillian Dickson

TODAY'S DATE _____

MEALS, BEVERAGES, SNACKS, AND SUPPLEMENTS

• Upon rising _____

• Before breakfast _____

• Breakfast _____

_____

• Midmorning snack _____

• Before lunch _____

• Lunch _____

_____

_____

_____

• 4 P.M. snack_____

• Before dinner_____

• Dinner_____

_____

_____

_____

• Midevening _____

HOURS SLEPT LAST NIGHT AND QUALITY OF SLEEP _____

_____

_____

_____

_____

EXERCISE _____

_____

_____

_____

HOW I IMPROVED FROM YESTERDAY _____

_____

_____

_____

HOW I FEEL PHYSICALLY _____

_____

_____

_____

_____

HOW I FEEL MENTALLY_____

_____

_____

_____

HOW I OVERCAME A CHALLENGE _____

_____

_____

_____

_____

WHAT I FEEL GRATEFUL FOR TODAY _____

_____

_____

_____

_____

WEEK 2: DAY 3

You had the power all along, my dear.

—*The Wizard of Oz*

TODAY'S DATE _____

MEALS, BEVERAGES, SNACKS, AND SUPPLEMENTS

• Upon rising _____

• Before breakfast _____

• Breakfast _____

_____

• Midmorning snack _____

• Before lunch _____

• Lunch _____

_____

_____

_____

• 4 P.M. snack_____

• Before dinner_____

• Dinner_____

_____

_____

_____

• Midevening _____

HOURS SLEPT LAST NIGHT AND QUALITY OF SLEEP _____

_____

_____

_____

_____

EXERCISE _____

_____

_____

_____

HOW I IMPROVED FROM YESTERDAY _____

_____

_____

_____

_____

HOW I FEEL PHYSICALLY _____

_____

_____

_____

_____

HOW I FEEL MENTALLY _____

_____

_____

_____

HOW I OVERCAME A CHALLENGE _____

_____

_____

_____

_____

WHAT I FEEL GRATEFUL FOR TODAY _____

_____

_____

_____

_____

_____

WEEK 2: DAY 4

Patience and determination alone are omnipotent. The slogan "press on" has solved and will always solve the problems of the human race.

—*Calvin Coolidge*

TODAY'S DATE _____

MEALS, BEVERAGES, SNACKS, AND SUPPLEMENTS

• Upon rising _____

• Before breakfast _____

• Breakfast _____

_____

• Midmorning snack _____

• Before lunch _____

• Lunch _____

_____

_____

_____

• 4 P.M. snack_____

• Before dinner_____

• Dinner_____

_____

_____

_____

• Midevening _____

HOURS SLEPT LAST NIGHT AND QUALITY OF SLEEP _____

_____

_____

_____

_____

EXERCISE _____

_____

_____

_____

HOW I IMPROVED FROM YESTERDAY _____

_____

_____

_____

_____

HOW I FEEL PHYSICALLY _____

_____

_____

_____

_____

HOW I FEEL MENTALLY_____

_____

_____

_____

HOW I OVERCAME A CHALLENGE _____

_____

_____

_____

_____

WHAT I FEEL GRATEFUL FOR TODAY _____

_____

_____

_____

_____

WEEK 2: DAY 5

If it doesn't challenge you, it won't change you.

—*Fred DeVito*

TODAY'S DATE _____

MEALS, BEVERAGES, SNACKS, AND SUPPLEMENTS

• Upon rising _____

• Before breakfast _____

• Breakfast _____

_____

• Midmorning snack _____

• Before lunch _____

• Lunch _____

_____

_____

_____

• 4 P.M. snack_____

• Before dinner_____

• Dinner_____

_____

_____

_____

• Midevening _____

HOURS SLEPT LAST NIGHT AND QUALITY OF SLEEP _____

_____

_____

_____

_____

EXERCISE _____

_____

_____

_____

HOW I IMPROVED FROM YESTERDAY _____

_____

_____

_____

HOW I FEEL PHYSICALLY _____

_____

_____

_____

HOW I FEEL MENTALLY_____

_____

_____

_____

HOW I OVERCAME A CHALLENGE _____

_____

_____

_____

WHAT I FEEL GRATEFUL FOR TODAY _____

_____

_____

_____

_____

WEEK 2: DAY 6

When you feel like quitting, think about why you started.
—*Anonymous*

TODAY'S DATE _____

MEALS, BEVERAGES, SNACKS, AND SUPPLEMENTS

• Upon rising _____

• Before breakfast _____

• Breakfast _____

_____

• Midmorning snack _____

• Before lunch _____

• Lunch _____

_____

_____

_____

• 4 P.M. snack_____

• Before dinner_____

• Dinner_____

_____

_____

_____

• Midevening _____

HOURS SLEPT LAST NIGHT AND QUALITY OF SLEEP _____

_____

_____

_____

_____

EXERCISE _____

_____

_____

_____

HOW I IMPROVED FROM YESTERDAY _____

_____

_____

_____

_____

HOW I FEEL PHYSICALLY _____

_____

_____

_____

_____

HOW I FEEL MENTALLY_____

_____

_____

_____

HOW I OVERCAME A CHALLENGE _____

_____

_____

_____

_____

WHAT I FEEL GRATEFUL FOR TODAY _____

_____

_____

_____

_____

_____

WEEK 2: DAY 7

Nothing can dim the light that shines from within.

—Maya Angelou

TODAY'S DATE _____

MEALS, BEVERAGES, SNACKS, AND SUPPLEMENTS

• Upon rising _____

• Before breakfast _____

• Breakfast _____

_____

• Midmorning snack _____

• Before lunch _____

• Lunch _____

_____

_____

_____

• 4 P.M. snack_____

• Before dinner_____

• Dinner_____

_____

_____

_____

• Midevening _____

HOURS SLEPT LAST NIGHT AND QUALITY OF SLEEP _____

_____

_____

_____

EXERCISE _____

_____

_____

_____

HOW I IMPROVED FROM YESTERDAY _____

_____

_____

_____

_____

HOW I FEEL PHYSICALLY _____

_____

_____

_____

_____

HOW I FEEL MENTALLY _____

_____

_____

_____

HOW I OVERCAME A CHALLENGE _____

_____

_____

_____

_____

WHAT I FEEL GRATEFUL FOR TODAY _____

_____

_____

_____

_____

_____

PREPARING FOR WEEK 3

Be patient with yourself as you evolve. Small, healthy choices make a difference in the long run!

—Anonymous

TODAY'S DATE _____

MY PHASE ____ GOAL ____ _____

_____

MEASUREMENTS

- Bust/Chest _____
- Waist _____
- Hips _____
- Thighs _____
- Weight _____

OVER THE PAST WEEK, HERE'S WHAT I'VE NOTICED ABOUT:

- The fit of my clothes_____
  _____
- My sleep patterns _____
  _____
  _____
- My energy level_____
  _____
  _____

- My emotional well-being _____

_____

_____

- My skin _____

_____

_____

MY BIGGEST STRUGGLE

_____

_____

_____

_____

MY BEST COMPLIMENT

_____

_____

_____

_____

MY PROUDEST MOMENT

_____

_____

_____

_____

THE BIGGEST CHALLENGES I ANTICIPATE THIS WEEK

_____

_____

_____

_____

A HABIT TAKES 21 DAYS TO FORM. MY HEALTHY HABIT (PHYSICAL OR SPRITIUAL) I'M BEGINNING OR CONTINUING TO DEVELOP THIS WEEK

_____

_____

_____

_____

_____

MY REWARD FOR A WEEK OF PROGRESS

_____

_____

_____

_____

MY MANTRA FOR THE WEEK

_____

_____

_____

_____

REMINDER: HOW REACHING MY GOAL WILL CHANGE MY LIFE

_____

_____

_____

_____

_____

WEEK 3: DAY 1

Life is a journey, and if you fall in love with the journey, you will be in love forever.

—Peter Hagerty

TODAY'S DATE _____

MEALS, BEVERAGES, SNACKS, AND SUPPLEMENTS

• Upon rising _____

• Before breakfast _____

• Breakfast _____

_____

• Midmorning snack _____

• Before lunch _____

• Lunch _____

_____

_____

_____

• 4 P.M. snack_____

• Before dinner_____

• Dinner_____

_____

_____

_____

• Midevening _____

HOURS SLEPT LAST NIGHT AND QUALITY OF SLEEP _____

_____

_____

_____

EXERCISE _____

_____

_____

_____

HOW I IMPROVED FROM YESTERDAY _____

_____

_____

_____

_____

HOW I FEEL PHYSICALLY _____

_____

_____

_____

_____

HOW I FEEL MENTALLY_____

_____

_____

_____

HOW I OVERCAME A CHALLENGE _____

_____

_____

_____

_____

WHAT I FEEL GRATEFUL FOR TODAY _____

_____

_____

_____

_____

WEEK 3: DAY 2

And now that you don't have to be perfect, you can be good.
—*John Steinbeck*

TODAY'S DATE _____

MEALS, BEVERAGES, SNACKS, AND SUPPLEMENTS

• Upon rising _____

• Before breakfast _____

• Breakfast _____

_____

• Midmorning snack _____

• Before lunch _____

• Lunch _____

_____

_____

_____

• 4 P.M. snack_____

• Before dinner_____

• Dinner_____

_____

_____

_____

• Midevening _____

HOURS SLEPT LAST NIGHT AND QUALITY OF SLEEP _____

_____

_____

_____

_____

EXERCISE _____

_____

_____

_____

HOW I IMPROVED FROM YESTERDAY _____

_____

_____

_____

_____

HOW I FEEL PHYSICALLY _____

_____

_____

_____

HOW I FEEL MENTALLY_____

_____

_____

_____

HOW I OVERCAME A CHALLENGE _____

_____

_____

_____

_____

WHAT I FEEL GRATEFUL FOR TODAY _____

_____

_____

_____

_____

WEEK 3: DAY 3

What matters most is how well you walk through the fire.
—Charles Bukowski

TODAY'S DATE _____

MEALS, BEVERAGES, SNACKS, AND SUPPLEMENTS

• Upon rising _____

• Before breakfast _____

• Breakfast _____

_____

• Midmorning snack _____

• Before lunch _____

• Lunch _____

_____

_____

_____

• 4 P.M. snack_____

• Before dinner_____

• Dinner_____

_____

_____

_____

• Midevening _____

HOURS SLEPT LAST NIGHT AND QUALITY OF SLEEP _____

_____

_____

_____

_____

EXERCISE _____

_____

_____

_____

HOW I IMPROVED FROM YESTERDAY _____

_____

_____

_____

HOW I FEEL PHYSICALLY _____

_____

_____

_____

_____

HOW I FEEL MENTALLY_____

_____

_____

_____

HOW I OVERCAME A CHALLENGE _____

_____

_____

_____

_____

WHAT I FEEL GRATEFUL FOR TODAY _____

_____

_____

_____

_____

_____

WEEK 3: DAY 4

> *I realized this week that I just cannot do it all. So, I will choose to do what I can, fabulously.*
>
> —*Clinton Kelly*

TODAY'S DATE _____

MEALS, BEVERAGES, SNACKS, AND SUPPLEMENTS

• Upon rising _____

• Before breakfast _____

• Breakfast _____

_____

• Midmorning snack _____

• Before lunch _____

• Lunch _____

_____

_____

_____

• 4 P.M. snack_____

• Before dinner_____

• Dinner_____

_____

_____

_____

• Midevening _____

HOURS SLEPT LAST NIGHT AND QUALITY OF SLEEP _____

_____

_____

_____

_____

EXERCISE _____

_____

_____

_____

HOW I IMPROVED FROM YESTERDAY _____

_____

_____

_____

_____

HOW I FEEL PHYSICALLY _____

_____

_____

_____

_____

HOW I FEEL MENTALLY_____

_____

_____

_____

HOW I OVERCAME A CHALLENGE _____

_____

_____

_____

_____

WHAT I FEEL GRATEFUL FOR TODAY _____

_____

_____

_____

_____

_____

WEEK 3: DAY 5

*I've been absolutely terrified every moment of my life—and
I've never let it keep me from doing a single thing I wanted
to do.*

—*Georgia O'Keeffe*

TODAY'S DATE _____

MEALS, BEVERAGES, SNACKS, AND SUPPLEMENTS

• Upon rising _____

• Before breakfast _____

• Breakfast _____

_____

• Midmorning snack _____

• Before lunch _____

• Lunch _____

_____

_____

_____

• 4 P.M. snack_____

• Before dinner_____

• Dinner_____

_____

_____

_____

• Midevening _____

HOURS SLEPT LAST NIGHT AND QUALITY OF SLEEP _____

_____

_____

_____

EXERCISE _____

_____

_____

_____

HOW I IMPROVED FROM YESTERDAY _____

_____

_____

_____

_____

HOW I FEEL PHYSICALLY _____

_____

_____

_____

_____

HOW I FEEL MENTALLY_____

_____

_____

_____

HOW I OVERCAME A CHALLENGE _____

_____

_____

_____

_____

WHAT I FEEL GRATEFUL FOR TODAY _____

_____

_____

_____

_____

WEEK 3: DAY 6

> *I'm not interested in competing with anyone. I hope we all make it.*
>
> —*Erica Cook*

TODAY'S DATE _____

MEALS, BEVERAGES, SNACKS, AND SUPPLEMENTS

• Upon rising _____

• Before breakfast _____

• Breakfast _____

_____

• Midmorning snack _____

• Before lunch _____

• Lunch _____

_____

_____

_____

• 4 P.M. snack_____

• Before dinner_____

• Dinner_____

_____

_____

_____

• Midevening _____

HOURS SLEPT LAST NIGHT AND QUALITY OF SLEEP _____

_____

_____

_____

_____

EXERCISE _____

_____

_____

_____

HOW I IMPROVED FROM YESTERDAY _____

_____

_____

_____

_____

HOW I FEEL PHYSICALLY _____

_____

_____

_____

_____

HOW I FEEL MENTALLY_____

_____

_____

_____

HOW I OVERCAME A CHALLENGE _____

_____

_____

_____

_____

WHAT I FEEL GRATEFUL FOR TODAY _____

_____

_____

_____

_____

WEEK 3: DAY 7

> *Authenticity is the daily practice of letting go of who we think we're supposed to be and embracing who we are.*
>
> —Brené Brown

TODAY'S DATE _____

MEALS, BEVERAGES, SNACKS, AND SUPPLEMENTS

• Upon rising _____

• Before breakfast _____

• Breakfast _____

_____

• Midmorning snack _____

• Before lunch _____

• Lunch _____

_____

_____

_____

• 4 P.M. snack_____

• Before dinner_____

• Dinner_____

_____

_____

_____

• Midevening _____

HOURS SLEPT LAST NIGHT AND QUALITY OF SLEEP _____

_____

_____

_____

_____

EXERCISE _____

_____

_____

_____

HOW I IMPROVED FROM YESTERDAY _____

_____

_____

_____

_____

HOW I FEEL PHYSICALLY _____

_____

_____

_____

_____

HOW I FEEL MENTALLY_____

_____

_____

_____

HOW I OVERCAME A CHALLENGE _____

_____

_____

_____

_____

WHAT I FEEL GRATEFUL FOR TODAY _____

_____

_____

_____

_____

_____

PREPARING FOR WEEK 4

Move out of your comfort zone. You can only grow if you are willing to feel awkward and uncomfortable when you try something new.

—BRIAN TRACY

TODAY'S DATE _____

MY PHASE _____ **GOAL** _____

_____

MEASUREMENTS

- Bust/Chest _____
- Waist _____
- Hips _____
- Thighs _____
- Weight _____

OVER THE PAST WEEK, HERE'S WHAT I'VE NOTICED ABOUT:

- The fit of my clothes _____

_____

- My sleep patterns _____

_____

_____

- My energy level _____

_____

_____

- My emotional well-being_____

  _____

  _____

- My skin_____

  _____

  _____

MY BIGGEST STRUGGLE

_____

_____

_____

_____

MY BEST COMPLIMENT

_____

_____

_____

_____

MY PROUDEST MOMENT

_____

_____

_____

_____

THE BIGGEST CHALLENGES I ANTICIPATE THIS WEEK

_____

_____

_____

_____

A HABIT TAKES 21 DAYS TO FORM. MY HEALTHY HABIT (PHYSICAL OR SPRITIUAL) I'M BEGINNING OR CONTINUING TO DEVELOP THIS WEEK

_____

_____

_____

_____

_____

MY REWARD FOR A WEEK OF PROGRESS

_____

_____

_____

_____

MY MANTRA FOR THE WEEK

_____

_____

_____

_____

REMINDER: HOW REACHING MY GOAL WILL CHANGE MY LIFE

_____

_____

_____

_____

_____

WEEK 4: DAY 1

The secret of change is to focus all of your energy not on fighting the old, but on building the new.

—Socrates

TODAY'S DATE _____

MEALS, BEVERAGES, SNACKS, AND SUPPLEMENTS

• Upon rising _____

• Before breakfast _____

• Breakfast _____

_____

• Midmorning snack _____

• Before lunch _____

• Lunch _____

_____

_____

_____

• 4 P.M. snack_____

• Before dinner_____

• Dinner_____

_____

_____

_____

• Midevening _____

HOURS SLEPT LAST NIGHT AND QUALITY OF SLEEP _____

_____

_____

_____

_____

EXERCISE _____

_____

_____

_____

HOW I IMPROVED FROM YESTERDAY _____

_____

_____

_____

_____

HOW I FEEL PHYSICALLY _____

_____

_____

_____

_____

HOW I FEEL MENTALLY _____

_____

_____

_____

HOW I OVERCAME A CHALLENGE _____

_____

_____

_____

_____

WHAT I FEEL GRATEFUL FOR TODAY _____

_____

_____

_____

_____

_____

WEEK 4: DAY 2

Your vision will become clear only when you look into your heart. Who looks outside, dreams. Who looks inside, awakens.

—Carl Jung

TODAY'S DATE _____

MEALS, BEVERAGES, SNACKS, AND SUPPLEMENTS

• Upon rising _____

• Before breakfast _____

• Breakfast _____

_____

• Midmorning snack _____

• Before lunch _____

• Lunch _____

_____

_____

_____

• 4 P.M. snack_____

• Before dinner_____

• Dinner_____

_____

_____

_____

• Midevening _____

HOURS SLEPT LAST NIGHT AND QUALITY OF SLEEP _____

_____

_____

_____

_____

EXERCISE _____

_____

_____

_____

HOW I IMPROVED FROM YESTERDAY _____

_____

_____

_____

_____

HOW I FEEL PHYSICALLY _____

_____

_____

_____

_____

HOW I FEEL MENTALLY_____

_____

_____

_____

HOW I OVERCAME A CHALLENGE _____

_____

_____

_____

_____

WHAT I FEEL GRATEFUL FOR TODAY _____

_____

_____

_____

_____

_____

WEEK 4: DAY 3

Your life is made of two dates and a dash. Make the most of the dash.

—Anonymous

TODAY'S DATE _____

MEALS, BEVERAGES, SNACKS, AND SUPPLEMENTS

• Upon rising _____

• Before breakfast _____

• Breakfast _____

_____

• Midmorning snack _____

• Before lunch _____

• Lunch _____

_____

_____

_____

• 4 P.M. snack_____

• Before dinner_____

• Dinner_____

_____

_____

_____

• Midevening _____

HOURS SLEPT LAST NIGHT AND QUALITY OF SLEEP _____

_____

_____

_____

_____

EXERCISE _____

_____

_____

_____

HOW I IMPROVED FROM YESTERDAY _____

_____

_____

_____

_____

HOW I FEEL PHYSICALLY _____

_____

_____

_____

_____

HOW I FEEL MENTALLY_____

_____

_____

_____

HOW I OVERCAME A CHALLENGE _____

_____

_____

_____

_____

WHAT I FEEL GRATEFUL FOR TODAY _____

_____

_____

_____

_____

WEEK 4: DAY 4

May your choices reflect your hopes, not your fears.
—Nelson Mandela

TODAY'S DATE _____

MEALS, BEVERAGES, SNACKS, AND SUPPLEMENTS

• Upon rising _____

• Before breakfast _____

• Breakfast _____

_____

• Midmorning snack _____

• Before lunch _____

• Lunch _____

_____

_____

_____

• 4 P.M. snack_____

• Before dinner_____

• Dinner_____

_____

_____

_____

• Midevening _____

HOURS SLEPT LAST NIGHT AND QUALITY OF SLEEP _____

_____

_____

_____

_____

EXERCISE _____

_____

_____

_____

HOW I IMPROVED FROM YESTERDAY _____

_____

_____

_____

_____

HOW I FEEL PHYSICALLY _____

_____

_____

_____

_____

HOW I FEEL MENTALLY _____

_____

_____

_____

_____

HOW I OVERCAME A CHALLENGE _____

_____

_____

_____

_____

WHAT I FEEL GRATEFUL FOR TODAY _____

_____

_____

_____

_____

WEEK 4: DAY 5

> *If you get the inside right, the outside will fall into place.*
> —Eckhart Tolle

TODAY'S DATE _____

MEALS, BEVERAGES, SNACKS, AND SUPPLEMENTS

• Upon rising _____

• Before breakfast _____

• Breakfast _____

_____

• Midmorning snack _____

• Before lunch _____

• Lunch _____

_____

_____

_____

• 4 P.M. snack_____

• Before dinner_____

• Dinner_____

_____

_____

_____

• Midevening _____

HOURS SLEPT LAST NIGHT AND QUALITY OF SLEEP _____

_____

_____

_____

_____

EXERCISE _____

_____

_____

_____

HOW I IMPROVED FROM YESTERDAY _____

_____

_____

_____

_____

HOW I FEEL PHYSICALLY _____

_____

_____

_____

_____

HOW I FEEL MENTALLY_____

_____

_____

_____

HOW I OVERCAME A CHALLENGE _____

_____

_____

_____

_____

WHAT I FEEL GRATEFUL FOR TODAY _____

_____

_____

_____

_____

WEEK 4: DAY 6

Our entire life consists ultimately in accepting ourselves as we are.

—*Jean Anouilh*

TODAY'S DATE _____

MEALS, BEVERAGES, SNACKS, AND SUPPLEMENTS

• Upon rising _____

• Before breakfast _____

• Breakfast _____

_____

• Midmorning snack _____

• Before lunch _____

• Lunch _____

_____

_____

_____

• 4 P.M. snack_____

• Before dinner_____

• Dinner_____

_____

_____

_____

• Midevening _____

HOURS SLEPT LAST NIGHT AND QUALITY OF SLEEP _____

_____

_____

_____

_____

EXERCISE _____

_____
_____
_____

HOW I IMPROVED FROM YESTERDAY _____

_____
_____
_____
_____

HOW I FEEL PHYSICALLY _____

_____
_____
_____
_____

HOW I FEEL MENTALLY_____

_____
_____
_____

HOW I OVERCAME A CHALLENGE _____

_____
_____
_____
_____

WHAT I FEEL GRATEFUL FOR TODAY _____

_____
_____
_____
_____
_____

WEEK 4: DAY 7

By being yourself you put something wonderful into the world that was not there before.

—*Edwin Elliot*

TODAY'S DATE _____

MEALS, BEVERAGES, SNACKS, AND SUPPLEMENTS

• Upon rising _____

• Before breakfast _____

• Breakfast _____

_____

• Midmorning snack _____

• Before lunch _____

• Lunch _____

_____

_____

_____

• 4 P.M. snack_____

• Before dinner_____

• Dinner_____

_____

_____

_____

• Midevening _____

HOURS SLEPT LAST NIGHT AND QUALITY OF SLEEP _____

_____

_____

_____

_____

Day 7

EXERCISE _____

_____

_____

_____

HOW I IMPROVED FROM YESTERDAY _____

_____

_____

_____

_____

HOW I FEEL PHYSICALLY _____

_____

_____

_____

_____

HOW I FEEL MENTALLY_____

_____

_____

_____

HOW I OVERCAME A CHALLENGE _____

_____

_____

_____

_____

WHAT I FEEL GRATEFUL FOR TODAY _____

_____

_____

_____

_____

_____

PREPARING FOR WEEK 5

Great things are done by a series of small things brought together.

—Vincent Van Gogh

TODAY'S DATE _____

MY PHASE _____ GOAL _____

_____

MEASUREMENTS

- Bust/Chest _____
- Waist _____
- Hips _____
- Thighs _____
- Weight _____

OVER THE PAST WEEK, HERE'S WHAT I'VE NOTICED ABOUT:

- The fit of my clothes_____

_____

- My sleep patterns _____

_____

_____

- My energy level_____

_____

_____

- My emotional well-being_____

  _____

  _____

- My skin_____

  _____

  _____

MY BIGGEST STRUGGLE

_____

_____

_____

_____

MY BEST COMPLIMENT

_____

_____

_____

_____

MY PROUDEST MOMENT

_____

_____

_____

_____

THE BIGGEST CHALLENGES I ANTICIPATE THIS WEEK

_____

_____

_____

_____

A HABIT TAKES 21 DAYS TO FORM. MY HEALTHY HABIT (PHYSICAL OR SPRITIUAL) I'M BEGINNING OR CONTINUING TO DEVELOP THIS WEEK

_____

_____

_____

_____

_____

MY REWARD FOR A WEEK OF PROGRESS

_____

_____

_____

_____

_____

MY MANTRA FOR THE WEEK

_____

_____

_____

_____

_____

REMINDER: HOW REACHING MY GOAL WILL CHANGE MY LIFE

_____

_____

_____

_____

_____

WEEK 5: DAY 1

I don't know a perfect person. I only know flawed people who are still worth loving.

—*John Green*

TODAY'S DATE _____

MEALS, BEVERAGES, SNACKS, AND SUPPLEMENTS

• Upon rising _____

• Before breakfast _____

• Breakfast _____

_____

• Midmorning snack _____

• Before lunch _____

• Lunch _____

_____

_____

_____

• 4 P.M. snack_____

• Before dinner_____

• Dinner_____

_____

_____

_____

• Midevening _____

HOURS SLEPT LAST NIGHT AND QUALITY OF SLEEP _____

_____

_____

_____

_____

EXERCISE _____

_____

_____

_____

HOW I IMPROVED FROM YESTERDAY _____

_____

_____

_____

HOW I FEEL PHYSICALLY _____

_____

_____

_____

_____

HOW I FEEL MENTALLY_____

_____

_____

_____

HOW I OVERCAME A CHALLENGE _____

_____

_____

_____

_____

WHAT I FEEL GRATEFUL FOR TODAY _____

_____

_____

_____

_____

WEEK 5: DAY 2

Attitude is the difference between an ordeal and an adventure.
—Bob Bitchin

TODAY'S DATE _____

MEALS, BEVERAGES, SNACKS, AND SUPPLEMENTS

• Upon rising _____

• Before breakfast _____

• Breakfast _____

_____

• Midmorning snack _____

• Before lunch _____

• Lunch _____

_____

_____

_____

• 4 P.M. snack_____

• Before dinner_____

• Dinner_____

_____

_____

_____

• Midevening _____

HOURS SLEPT LAST NIGHT AND QUALITY OF SLEEP _____

_____

_____

_____

_____

EXERCISE _____

_____

_____

_____

HOW I IMPROVED FROM YESTERDAY _____

_____

_____

_____

_____

HOW I FEEL PHYSICALLY _____

_____

_____

_____

_____

HOW I FEEL MENTALLY _____

_____

_____

_____

HOW I OVERCAME A CHALLENGE _____

_____

_____

_____

_____

WHAT I FEEL GRATEFUL FOR TODAY _____

_____

_____

_____

_____

_____

WEEK 5: DAY 3

In optimism there is magic. In pessimism there is nothing.
—Abraham Hicks

TODAY'S DATE _____

MEALS, BEVERAGES, SNACKS, AND SUPPLEMENTS

• Upon rising _____

• Before breakfast _____

• Breakfast _____

_____

• Midmorning snack _____

• Before lunch _____

• Lunch _____

_____

_____

_____

• 4 P.M. snack_____

• Before dinner_____

• Dinner_____

_____

_____

_____

• Midevening _____

HOURS SLEPT LAST NIGHT AND QUALITY OF SLEEP _____

_____

_____

_____

_____

EXERCISE _____

_____

_____

_____

HOW I IMPROVED FROM YESTERDAY _____

_____

_____

_____

_____

HOW I FEEL PHYSICALLY _____

_____

_____

_____

_____

HOW I FEEL MENTALLY _____

_____

_____

_____

HOW I OVERCAME A CHALLENGE _____

_____

_____

_____

_____

WHAT I FEEL GRATEFUL FOR TODAY _____

_____

_____

_____

_____

_____

WEEK 5: DAY 4

When life is sweet, say thank you and celebrate. When life is bitter, say thank you and grow.

—*Shauna Niequist*

TODAY'S DATE _____

MEALS, BEVERAGES, SNACKS, AND SUPPLEMENTS

• Upon rising _____

• Before breakfast _____

• Breakfast _____

_____

• Midmorning snack _____

• Before lunch _____

• Lunch _____

_____

_____

_____

• 4 P.M. snack_____

• Before dinner_____

• Dinner_____

_____

_____

_____

• Midevening _____

HOURS SLEPT LAST NIGHT AND QUALITY OF SLEEP _____

_____

_____

_____

_____

EXERCISE _____

_____

_____

_____

HOW I IMPROVED FROM YESTERDAY _____

_____

_____

_____

_____

HOW I FEEL PHYSICALLY _____

_____

_____

_____

_____

HOW I FEEL MENTALLY_____

_____

_____

_____

HOW I OVERCAME A CHALLENGE _____

_____

_____

_____

WHAT I FEEL GRATEFUL FOR TODAY _____

_____

_____

_____

_____

_____

WEEK 5: DAY 5

> *I survived because the fire inside me burned brighter than the fire around me.*
>
> —*Joshua Graham*

TODAY'S DATE _____

MEALS, BEVERAGES, SNACKS, AND SUPPLEMENTS

• Upon rising _____

• Before breakfast _____

• Breakfast _____

_____

• Midmorning snack _____

• Before lunch _____

• Lunch _____

_____

_____

_____

• 4 P.M. snack_____

• Before dinner_____

• Dinner_____

_____

_____

_____

• Midevening _____

HOURS SLEPT LAST NIGHT AND QUALITY OF SLEEP _____

_____

_____

_____

_____

EXERCISE _____

_____

_____

_____

HOW I IMPROVED FROM YESTERDAY _____

_____

_____

_____

_____

HOW I FEEL PHYSICALLY _____

_____

_____

_____

_____

HOW I FEEL MENTALLY_____

_____

_____

_____

HOW I OVERCAME A CHALLENGE _____

_____

_____

_____

_____

WHAT I FEEL GRATEFUL FOR TODAY _____

_____

_____

_____

_____

WEEK 5: DAY 6

You'll turn out ordinary if you're not careful.

—Ann Brashes

TODAY'S DATE _____

MEALS, BEVERAGES, SNACKS, AND SUPPLEMENTS

• Upon rising _____

• Before breakfast _____

• Breakfast _____

_____

• Midmorning snack _____

• Before lunch _____

• Lunch _____

_____

_____

_____

• 4 P.M. snack_____

• Before dinner_____

• Dinner_____

_____

_____

_____

• Midevening _____

HOURS SLEPT LAST NIGHT AND QUALITY OF SLEEP _____

_____

_____

_____

_____

EXERCISE _____

_____

_____

_____

HOW I IMPROVED FROM YESTERDAY _____

_____

_____

_____

_____

HOW I FEEL PHYSICALLY _____

_____

_____

_____

_____

HOW I FEEL MENTALLY_____

_____

_____

_____

HOW I OVERCAME A CHALLENGE _____

_____

_____

_____

_____

WHAT I FEEL GRATEFUL FOR TODAY _____

_____

_____

_____

_____

WEEK 5: DAY 7

Close your eyes and imagine the best version of you possible. That's who you really are. Let go of any part of you that doesn't believe it.

—C. Assaad

TODAY'S DATE _____

MEALS, BEVERAGES, SNACKS, AND SUPPLEMENTS

• Upon rising _____

• Before breakfast _____

• Breakfast _____

_____

• Midmorning snack _____

• Before lunch _____

• Lunch _____

_____

_____

_____

• 4 P.M. snack_____

• Before dinner_____

• Dinner_____

_____

_____

_____

• Midevening _____

HOURS SLEPT LAST NIGHT AND QUALITY OF SLEEP _____

_____

_____

_____

_____

EXERCISE _____

_____

_____

_____

HOW I IMPROVED FROM YESTERDAY _____

_____

_____

_____

_____

HOW I FEEL PHYSICALLY _____

_____

_____

_____

_____

HOW I FEEL MENTALLY _____

_____

_____

_____

HOW I OVERCAME A CHALLENGE _____

_____

_____

_____

_____

WHAT I FEEL GRATEFUL FOR TODAY _____

_____

_____

_____

_____

_____

PREPARING FOR WEEK 6

One of the greatest weaknesses in most of us is our lack of faith in ourselves. One of our common failings is to depreciate our tremendous worth.

—L. Tom Perry

TODAY'S DATE _____

MY PHASE _____ GOAL _____

_____

MEASUREMENTS

* Bust/Chest _____
* Waist _____
* Hips _____
* Thighs _____
* Weight _____

OVER THE PAST WEEK, HERE'S WHAT I'VE NOTICED ABOUT:

* The fit of my clothes_____

_____

* My sleep patterns _____

_____

_____

* My energy level_____

_____

_____

- My emotional well-being_____

  _____

  _____

- My skin_____

  _____

  _____

MY BIGGEST STRUGGLE

_____

_____

_____

_____

MY BEST COMPLIMENT

_____

_____

_____

_____

MY PROUDEST MOMENT

_____

_____

_____

_____

THE BIGGEST CHALLENGES I ANTICIPATE THIS WEEK

_____

_____

_____

_____

A HABIT TAKES 21 DAYS TO FORM. MY HEALTHY HABIT (PHYSICAL OR SPRITIUAL) I'M BEGINNING OR CONTINUING TO DEVELOP THIS WEEK

_____

_____

_____

_____

_____

MY REWARD FOR A WEEK OF PROGRESS

_____

_____

_____

_____

MY MANTRA FOR THE WEEK

_____

_____

_____

_____

REMINDER: HOW REACHING MY GOAL WILL CHANGE MY LIFE

_____

_____

_____

_____

WEEK 6: DAY 1

Perfect is empty. Boring. Vapid. Exhausting. Be interesting.
Be interested. Be anything except on a quest for perfect.
—*Victoria Erickson*

TODAY'S DATE _____

MEALS, BEVERAGES, SNACKS, AND SUPPLEMENTS

• Upon rising _____

• Before breakfast _____

• Breakfast _____

_____

• Midmorning snack _____

• Before lunch _____

• Lunch _____

_____

_____

_____

• 4 P.M. snack_____

• Before dinner_____

• Dinner_____

_____

_____

_____

• Midevening _____

HOURS SLEPT LAST NIGHT AND QUALITY OF SLEEP _____

_____

_____

_____

_____

EXERCISE _____

_____

_____

_____

HOW I IMPROVED FROM YESTERDAY _____

_____

_____

_____

_____

HOW I FEEL PHYSICALLY _____

_____

_____

_____

HOW I FEEL MENTALLY_____

_____

_____

_____

HOW I OVERCAME A CHALLENGE _____

_____

_____

_____

WHAT I FEEL GRATEFUL FOR TODAY _____

_____

_____

_____

_____

_____

WEEK 6: DAY 2

Fall in love with taking care of yourself. Mind. Body. Spirit.
                                                    —*Anonymous*

TODAY'S DATE _____

MEALS, BEVERAGES, SNACKS, AND SUPPLEMENTS

• Upon rising _____

• Before breakfast _____

• Breakfast _____

_____

• Midmorning snack _____

• Before lunch _____

• Lunch _____

_____

_____

_____

• 4 P.M. snack_____

• Before dinner_____

• Dinner_____

_____

_____

_____

• Midevening _____

HOURS SLEPT LAST NIGHT AND QUALITY OF SLEEP _____

_____

_____

_____

_____

EXERCISE _____

_____

_____

_____

HOW I IMPROVED FROM YESTERDAY _____

_____

_____

_____

_____

HOW I FEEL PHYSICALLY _____

_____

_____

_____

_____

HOW I FEEL MENTALLY_____

_____

_____

_____

HOW I OVERCAME A CHALLENGE _____

_____

_____

_____

_____

WHAT I FEEL GRATEFUL FOR TODAY _____

_____

_____

_____

_____

_____

WEEK 6: DAY 3

I have already lost touch with a couple of people I used to be.
—Joan Didion

TODAY'S DATE _____

MEALS, BEVERAGES, SNACKS, AND SUPPLEMENTS

• Upon rising _____

• Before breakfast _____

• Breakfast _____

_____

• Midmorning snack _____

• Before lunch _____

• Lunch _____

_____

_____

_____

• 4 P.M. snack_____

• Before dinner_____

• Dinner_____

_____

_____

_____

• Midevening _____

HOURS SLEPT LAST NIGHT AND QUALITY OF SLEEP _____

_____

_____

_____

_____

EXERCISE _____

_____

_____

_____

HOW I IMPROVED FROM YESTERDAY _____

_____

_____

_____

_____

HOW I FEEL PHYSICALLY _____

_____

_____

_____

_____

HOW I FEEL MENTALLY_____

_____

_____

_____

HOW I OVERCAME A CHALLENGE _____

_____

_____

_____

_____

WHAT I FEEL GRATEFUL FOR TODAY _____

_____

_____

_____

_____

_____

WEEK 6: DAY 4

It takes courage to grow up and become who you really are.
—*E. E. Cummings*

TODAY'S DATE _____

MEALS, BEVERAGES, SNACKS, AND SUPPLEMENTS

• Upon rising _____

• Before breakfast _____

• Breakfast _____

_____

• Midmorning snack _____

• Before lunch _____

• Lunch _____

_____

_____

_____

• 4 P.M. snack_____

• Before dinner_____

• Dinner_____

_____

_____

_____

• Midevening _____

HOURS SLEPT LAST NIGHT AND QUALITY OF SLEEP _____

_____

_____

_____

_____

EXERCISE _____

_____

_____

_____

HOW I IMPROVED FROM YESTERDAY _____

_____

_____

_____

HOW I FEEL PHYSICALLY _____

_____

_____

_____

HOW I FEEL MENTALLY_____

_____

_____

_____

HOW I OVERCAME A CHALLENGE _____

_____

_____

_____

WHAT I FEEL GRATEFUL FOR TODAY _____

_____

_____

_____

_____

WEEK 6: DAY 5

Don't live the same year 75 times and call it a life.

—*Robin Sharma*

TODAY'S DATE _____

MEALS, BEVERAGES, SNACKS, AND SUPPLEMENTS

• Upon rising _____

• Before breakfast _____

• Breakfast _____

_____

• Midmorning snack _____

• Before lunch _____

• Lunch _____

_____

_____

_____

• 4 P.M. snack_____

• Before dinner_____

• Dinner_____

_____

_____

_____

• Midevening _____

HOURS SLEPT LAST NIGHT AND QUALITY OF SLEEP _____

_____

_____

_____

_____

EXERCISE _____

_____

_____

_____

HOW I IMPROVED FROM YESTERDAY _____

_____

_____

_____

_____

HOW I FEEL PHYSICALLY _____

_____

_____

_____

_____

HOW I FEEL MENTALLY_____

_____

_____

_____

HOW I OVERCAME A CHALLENGE _____

_____

_____

_____

_____

WHAT I FEEL GRATEFUL FOR TODAY _____

_____

_____

_____

_____

_____

WEEK 6: DAY 6

Hope is like the sun, which, as we journey toward it, casts the shadow of our burden behind us.

—*Samuel Smiles*

TODAY'S DATE _____

MEALS, BEVERAGES, SNACKS, AND SUPPLEMENTS

• Upon rising _____

• Before breakfast _____

• Breakfast _____

_____

• Midmorning snack _____

• Before lunch _____

• Lunch _____

_____

_____

_____

• 4 P.M. snack_____

• Before dinner_____

• Dinner_____

_____

_____

_____

• Midevening _____

HOURS SLEPT LAST NIGHT AND QUALITY OF SLEEP _____

_____

_____

_____

_____

EXERCISE _____

_____

_____

_____

HOW I IMPROVED FROM YESTERDAY _____

_____

_____

_____

_____

HOW I FEEL PHYSICALLY _____

_____

_____

_____

_____

HOW I FEEL MENTALLY_____

_____

_____

_____

HOW I OVERCAME A CHALLENGE _____

_____

_____

_____

_____

WHAT I FEEL GRATEFUL FOR TODAY _____

_____

_____

_____

_____

WEEK 6: DAY 7

I am the me I choose to be.

—*Sidney Poitier*

TODAY'S DATE _____

MEALS, BEVERAGES, SNACKS, AND SUPPLEMENTS

• Upon rising _____

• Before breakfast _____

• Breakfast _____

_____

• Midmorning snack _____

• Before lunch _____

• Lunch _____

_____

_____

_____

• 4 P.M. snack_____

• Before dinner_____

• Dinner_____

_____

_____

_____

• Midevening _____

HOURS SLEPT LAST NIGHT AND QUALITY OF SLEEP _____

_____

_____

_____

_____

EXERCISE _____

_____

_____

_____

HOW I IMPROVED FROM YESTERDAY _____

_____

_____

_____

_____

HOW I FEEL PHYSICALLY _____

_____

_____

_____

_____

HOW I FEEL MENTALLY_____

_____

_____

_____

HOW I OVERCAME A CHALLENGE _____

_____

_____

_____

_____

WHAT I FEEL GRATEFUL FOR TODAY _____

_____

_____

_____

_____

PREPARING FOR MY NEW FAT FLUSH LIFESTYLE

Everything you want is on the other side of fear.
— JACK CANFIELD

MEASUREMENTS

- Bust/Chest _____

- Waist _____

- Hips _____

- Thighs _____

- Weight _____

OVER THE PAST WEEK, HERE'S WHAT I'VE NOTICED ABOUT:

- The fit of my clothes_____

  _____

- My sleep patterns _____

  _____

  _____

- My energy level_____

  _____

  _____

- My emotional well-being_____

  _____

  _____

- My skin_____

  _____

MY BIGGEST STRUGGLE

_____

_____

_____

_____

MY BEST COMPLIMENT

_____

_____

_____

_____

MY PROUDEST MOMENT

_____

_____

_____

_____

MOVING FORWARD

**THE BIGGEST CHALLENGES I ANTICIPATE WITH STAYING ON COURSE
WITH MY NEW LIFESTYLE**

_____

_____

_____

_____

_____

_____

_____

THE NEW HEALTHY HABITS I'VE FORMED

_____

_____

_____

_____

_____

MY REWARD FOR THE PROGRESS I'VE MADE

_____

_____

_____

_____

MY NEW MANTRA FOR LIFE

_____

_____

_____

_____

HOW I WILL STAY ON TRACK

_____

_____

_____

_____

_____

_____

WHAT I WILL DO IF I GET OFF TRACK

_____

_____

_____

_____

_____

_____

HOW MY LIFE HAS CHANGED

_____

_____

_____

_____

_____

Notes

About the Author

Ann Louise Gittleman, PhD, CNS, is undisputedly the First Lady of Nutrition. As a nutritional visionary and health pioneer, she has fearlessly stood on the front lines of diet and detox, the environment, and women's health. *Self* magazine describes her as one of the Top Ten Notable Nutritionists in the United States, and thousands of nutritionists, health coaches, and practitioners have benefited from her work.

Years before the Paleo, ketogenic, and vegan diet trends, in her first book, *Beyond Pritikin* (1988), Ann Louise was the very first to proclaim that obesity and diabetes were caused by a lack of the right type of fat and an excess of the wrong kind of carbohydrates, including gluten-rich grain. She was also the first nutritionist to write about the perils of gluten and discuss the blood-type theory in 1996, boldly stating, in her book *Your Body Knows Best*, that one diet may not be right for everyone.

She has also been a tireless crusader for women by offering natural solutions to menopause and perimenopausal symptoms, decades before anybody else, in her award-winning *Super Nutrition for Women*, as well as *Super Nutrition for Menopause* and her *New York Times* bestseller *Before the Change*.

She then revolutionized dieting in the first edition of *The Fat Flush Plan*—an international bestseller—by proclaiming that the liver was the body's primary fat-burning organ (and detoxifier).

Most recently, she led the charge against the hidden hazards of cell phones, iPads, smart meters, and WiFi in her groundbreaking book *Zapped*.

She has appeared on *20/20*, *Dr. Phil*, *The View*, *Good Morning America*, *Extra!*, *FitTV*, and *The Early Show*. In addition, her work has been featured on ABC, CNN, PBS, CBS, NBC, MSNBC, CBN, Fox News, and the BBC.

She has served as a celebrity spokesperson and formula developer for many of the leading companies in the health foods and network marketing industry. Her work has been featured in a myriad of national publications including *Time*, *Newsweek*, *Glamour*, and the *New York Times*.

ENGAGING HEALTH

Today she continues to dedicate herself to carving out new landmarks in functional and integrative medicine with her latest e-book, *Eat Fat, Lose Weight*. She is a popular speaker on Internet summits and is actively involved with videos and her blog. Her expert advice often appears in *First for Women* magazine, where she was the nutrition columnist for more than 10 years.

In 2016 Ann Louise was presented with the Humanitarian Award from the Cancer Control Society. She currently sits on the Advisory Board for the International Institute for Building-Biology & Ecology, the Nutritional Therapy Association, Inc., and Clear Passage, Inc.

Connect with Ann Louise at www.annlouise.com, www.fatflush.com, and facebook.com/annlouisegittleman.

Books from Award-Winning Pioneer Nutritionalist Ann Louise Gittleman, PH.D, C.N.S.

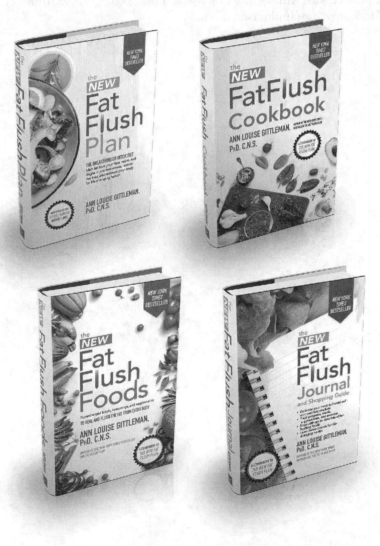